Praise for *What I Thought I Knew*
by Alice Eve Cohen

"Cohen is first and foremost a performer—a writer and actor of one-woman plays—so she knows how to build tension to a climax. Her easy intimacy when recounting the events of a pivotal year of her life is amazing."   —*BookPage*

"Her witty, dramatic story builds suspense up to the final page."
                                                                                   —*More*

"I found Cohen's fast-paced and intimate storytelling drawing me in and compelling me to be a part of her journey. It's almost like sitting with an especially candid friend and listening to her story."
                        —Roxanne J. Coady, Women on the Web (wowOwow.com)

"If you've ever found yourself or a loved one in the strange terrain where ethics and practical thought conflict, this will clarify and inspire."   —*Remedy*

"I could not put this book down. I got to the last pages, and I had tears in my eyes. It is a remarkable story."
                                            —Harry Smith, CBS, *The Early Show*

"It is rare for a memoir about motherhood to read like a thriller, but *What I Thought I Knew* . . . is just that. The book is fascinating, brutally honest, and very funny."   —Annie Pleshette Murphy, *ABC News Now*

"By turns black comedy, Kafkaesque nightmare, medical mystery, and crisis of faith, *What I Thought I Knew* is ultimately a love story. Blessed with a witty, unsentimental, utterly human voice, Alice Eve Cohen has taken what might have been a personal catastrophe and turned it into a memoir of astonishing candor."
                        —Donald Margulies, author of *Dinner with Friends,* winner
                           of the Pulitzer Prize for Drama

"A hell of a well told story—a book you won't put down. I loved every word."   —Abigail Thomas, author of *A Three Dog Life*

"This wonderful, uplifting book is about facing life on life's terms. . . . Many people will see themselves reflected in this fascinating story."
                        —Winnie Holzman, book writer for the musical *Wicked*

"Alice Eve Cohen is a true storyteller. . . . Her smart, intimate, quirky book is not so much a memoir as it is a tale: the question isn't just 'Who am I?' but 'What kind of universe is this?'"
—Joan Wickersham, author of National Book Award finalist *The Suicide Index*

"Alice writes with humor, guts, and honesty, while spinning her unbelievable yet true tale like a master. I laughed; I cried. I crashed with her losses; I soared with her triumphs. And I was gripped through every twist and turn. Alice Eve Cohen is my new hero. I aspire to look at my own life's challenges with her kind of ferocity and heartfelt wit." —Jacquelyn Reingold, playwright and writer for HBO's *In Treatment*

"Candid, brave, and heartbreakingly funny. As her situation goes from bad to worse to unthinkable, Cohen not only survives but triumphs with integrity, hope, and a sense of humor that is matched only by her courage."
—Patricia McCormick, author of National Book Award finalist *Sold*

"A true page-turner: a compelling and utterly unique human journey told with ruthless honesty and humor. All I kept thinking was 'what a woman!'" —Christine Baranski, Emmy-, Tony-, SAG-, and Drama Desk Award–winning actress

"Captivating, beautifully written, inspiring, *What I Thought I Knew* should be read by every medical school student."
—Jeffrey Trilling, MD, associate professor and chair, department of family medicine, Stony Brook School of Medicine

"This remarkable book . . . feels like an intimate conversation about the most earth-shaking moments in a woman's life. . . . After reading this book, we may discover what we thought we knew and what we believe we know today." —Maxine Greene

"I love this book. I read it in two straight days and made everyone I know read it too. Then they ll started to drive me crazy by calling to read me the funniest line, or the most touching."
—Anne Lamott, author of *Bird by Bird* and *Grace (Eventually)*

PENGUIN BOOKS

WHAT I THOUGHT I KNEW

Alice Eve Cohen is a playwright, solo theater artist, and memoirist. She has written for Nickelodeon and PBS and received fellowships and grants from the New York State Council on the Arts and the National Endowment for the Arts. *What I Thought I Knew* won *Elle*'s 2009 Grand Prix for nonfiction and was featured by *O, The Oprah Magazine* as one of the 25 Best Books of Summer. She teaches at The New School in New York City.

what i
thought
i knew

Alice Eve Cohen

PENGUIN BOOKS

PENGUIN BOOKS

Published by the Penguin Group
Penguin Group (USA) Inc., 375 Hudson Street, New York, New York 10014, U.S.A. • Penguin Group
(Canada), 90 Eglinton Avenue East, Suite 700, Toronto, Ontario, Canada M4P 2Y3 (a division of Pearson
Penguin Canada Inc.) • Penguin Books Ltd, 80 Strand, London WC2R 0RL, England • Penguin Ireland,
25 St Stephen's Green, Dublin 2, Ireland (a division of Penguin Books Ltd) • Penguin Group (Australia),
250 Camberwell Road, Camberwell, Victoria 3124, Australia (a division of Pearson Australia Group
Pty Ltd) • Penguin Books India Pvt Ltd, 11 Community Centre, Panchsheel Park, New Delhi – 110 017,
India • Penguin Group (NZ), 67 Apollo Drive, Rosedale, North Shore 0632, New Zealand (a division
of Pearson New Zealand Ltd) • Penguin Books (South Africa) (Pty) Ltd, 24 Sturdee Avenue,
Rosebank, Johannesburg 2196, South Africa

Penguin Books Ltd, Registered Offices: 80 Strand, London WC2R 0RL, England

First published in the United States of America by Viking Penguin,
a member of Penguin Group (USA) Inc. 2009
Published in Penguin Books 2010

10   9   8   7   6   5   4   3   2   1

Grateful acknowledgment is made for permission to reprint an excerpt from *Dust Tracks on a Road* by Zora
Neale Hurston. Copyright 1942 by Zora Neale Hurston, copyright renewed © 1970 by John C. Hurston.
Reprinted by permission of HarperCollins Publishers.

The Brocaded Slipper and Other Vietnamese Tales by Lynette Dyer Vuong; text copyright 1982 by Lynette Dyer
Vuong; used by permission of HarperCollins Publishers.

THE LIBRARY OF CONGRESS HAS CATALOGED THE HARDCOVER EDITION AS FOLLOWS:
Cohen, Alice Eve.
What I thought I knew / Alice Eve Cohen.
p.   cm.
ISBN 978-0-670-02095-9 (hc.)
ISBN 978-0-14-311765-0 (pbk.)
1. Motherhood—United States—Case studies.   2. Mother and child—United States—Case studies.
3. Pregnancy, unwanted—United States—Case studies.   4. Fetal growth retardation—United States—Case
studies.   5. Birth weight, Low—United States—Case studies.   6. Cohen, Alice Eve.   7. Cohen, Alice Eve—
Family.   8. Parents of children with disabilities—United States—Biography.   9. Mothers and daughters—
United States—Biography.   10. Jewish women—United States—Biography.   I. Title.
HQ759.C644 2009
306.874'3092—dc22
[B] 2008051576

Printed in the United States of America
Set in Life • Designed by Alissa Amell

Penguin is committed to publishing works of quality and integrity.
In that spirit, we are proud to offer this book to our readers;
however, the story, the experiences, and the words
are the author's alone.

For my wonderful family

author's note

All the events in this book actually occurred. As this is a memoir, my telling of the events is filtered through the lens of memory and emotion, and altered by the passage of time. I've changed the names and identifying details of some people in this book to protect their privacy. Conversations and dialogues have been modified by memory, and sometimes intentionally compressed and reshaped for narrative purposes. My intent throughout the book is to re-create for the reader the story as I experienced it in the moment, and in the state of mind I was in at each stage in the journey. This is how I remember my life during this period of time.

There is no agony like bearing an untold story inside of you.

—Zora Neale Hurston

Contents

ACT I

Unbridled Good Fortune

Scene 1

Stage Fright

This was going to be a solo show. That's what I do. I write and perform solo plays. Dramatic tales with multiple characters, for adults. Comic plays and folktales, for children. I've performed for half a million people, in tiny theaters and high-tech performance spaces, in international theater festivals and school cafeterias, on four continents.

I rarely get stage fright. But the thought of performing this story in front of an audience was like willingly entering my recurrent dream—the one where I am standing under a blinding spotlight on a rickety proscenium stage. I face the audience, open my mouth to speak, and realize: 1) I can't remember my lines; 2) There is a marching band entering the theater; 3) I'm naked. Shouting over the brass section, I stammer and blurt out improvisations, hoping my lines will come back to me before the audience showers me with rotten vegetables, but the band drowns me out. As they approach the stage, I see that the musicians are wild animals in military dress. I wake in a sweat.

On Friday, the eve of the Jewish New Year, September 10,

1999, I was rushed to Lenox Hill Hospital for an emergency CAT scan. "I'm here with your patient," said the radiologist on the phone to my doctor. "She appears to be in shock."

I sat down to write this story as a solo show, but I got stage fright and couldn't write anything for years.

Seven years later, on Friday, the eve of the Jewish New Year, 2006, I started to write. Unexpectedly. Urgently.

I won't be performing this story. In a book I am just as naked, lit under as unforgiving a spotlight, but I'm willing to divulge these secrets for one reader at a time. I've been writing as fast as I can, without telling anybody. For fear that I'll stop. For fear that the Evil Eye will catch up with me. Again.

Scene 2

Unbridled Good Fortune

This is the happiest I've been in years. As if in a perpetual state of inebriation, I laugh for no reason. I celebrate the end of the decade and the millennium.

The first half of the nineties was less celebratory. Infertility. Divorce from Brad after thirteen years together. A custody battle for our three-year-old adopted daughter, Julia. The loneliness of single parenthood. The exhausting discipline of raising Julia on my minimal, freelance income. The fear of raising a child in my crime-ridden building. Before taking Julia out for a walk in her stroller, I had to look through the peephole to make sure my drug-dealing neighbor wasn't starting a gunfight with an unruly client.

In the spring of 1999, I indulge in the pleasurable delusion of eternal youth. Michael, my fiancé, is ten years younger. I'm forty-four. He's thirty-four, but he looks like a college kid, with his wayward curly hair, earnest blue gray eyes, baggy jeans, and thread-bare T-shirt, cradling his guitar and singing the song he wrote last night instead of sleeping. He's smart, funny, cynical, affectionate. He'll never grow up, and as long as I'm with him, neither will I.

We met three years earlier at a children's theater conference, where we were both performing solo plays. He drove me home, came back for dinner the next night, and spent the night. Because of our age difference, we had no expectations that our fling would develop into anything more. Because we had no expectations, we shed our armor. When we shed our armor, we fell in love.

Michael grew up in New Orleans, and was the only one in his conservative, devout Lutheran family who'd ever moved north of the Mason-Dixon Line. After his family recovered from hearing that he was dating a Jewish New Yorker—a divorced, single mom, ten years his senior—they teased him about acquiring an instant family. Michael had always preferred to let his life happen to him, rather than plan it.

Michael was nearly penniless, by design. Money didn't interest him. His professional passion was creating theater with kids in the country's poorest communities—impoverished school districts in southern Appalachia, children of Mexican migrant workers in El Paso, Texas—where he slept on the sofas of local families and barely broke even. He paid the rent with his more remunerative corporate theater jobs.

From the first day they met, Michael and Julia, then five years old, hit it off. I left them in the apartment while I picked up dinner from the Cuban Chinese restaurant down the block. When I returned with the yellow rice and black beans, they were sitting on the floor of Julia's room inventing an elaborate story, which they animated with Julia's stuffed animals and a talking basket. When he moved in with us a year later, he brought everything he owned: hundreds of books, a crate of handmade masks and puppets, two guitars, and the futon he'd carried with him to the fourteen places he'd lived since graduating from the University of Virginia.

In the spring of 1999, Michael and Julia, now eight, are great friends. He wants to raise Julia with me, but he doesn't want to have more children. Neither do I.

Brad moved to Los Angeles when Julia was five. Three thousand miles has done wonders for our relationship. Julia keeps a photo of Brad by her bed, a formal performance portrait: Tall and thin, with intensely dark eyes and thick black hair, he is wearing a tuxedo and conducting the final, wrenching movement of Mahler's Ninth Symphony. Julia visits him in LA on holidays.

I am in school, finishing up my MFA in writing for children at The New School University, an easy subway commute from our Upper West Side apartment to the Greenwich Village campus. Because classes are at night, I can continue my freelance work during the day. In exchange for The New School's reasonable tuition, I'm getting the degree I need to teach college, and the luxury of two years of creative immersion. When Julia was younger, I couldn't afford to write anything that didn't pay the bills.

I love being in school, and I'm writing day and night. I still dress like I did as a Princeton student in the midseventies, half my life ago: jeans and a T-shirt, my long dark hair (now with a few renegade grays) worn loose. After class, I drink beer with my grad school friends at Cedar Tavern, a ragtag Greenwich Village bar with dark paneling, cheap beer, and an infamous history of

ill-behaved artists—Jack Kerouac was thrown out in the forties
for pissing in an ashtray, Jackson Pollock in the fifties for ripping
the door off the men's room.

One night, my friend Dylan catches my eye when he enters the
classroom. Gay, universally flirtatious, and mercilessly beautiful,
Dylan has a habit of breaking his professors' hearts—dating,
breaking up with, and intellectually disabling otherwise erudite
teachers. Dylan kneels in front of my chair, gazes into my eyes,
and whispers, "You're pregnant, Alice, aren't you?"

"No!"

"Yes you are. You have that erotic glow that only a pregnant
woman has."

"I'm not pregnant."

He examines me more closely and whispers, "Then you had
really hot sex last night."

In fact, Michael and I did have hot sex last night, after he
proposed to me and I said yes. My erotic glow is showing! In this
deliriously happy spring, after my postdivorce winter that lasted
half a decade, I have found the fountain of youth.

My unbridled good fortune gallops on at reckless speed.

My agent books a full season of performances of my solo theater works, in humble and exalted venues throughout the East
Coast, lucrative and fun work.

The manager of my building evicts the drug dealers and hires
a doorman.

The New School hires me to teach solo theater, starting in the
fall.

My part-time editing job, plus the new part-time teaching gig, gives me a steady freelance income and a flexible schedule.

We can afford a family vacation—Michael, Julia, and I are going to Italy in August.

For the first time in years, I have time to write, I don't have to buy clothes at the thrift store, I'm not worried about making rent. I can breathe.

I'm in love.

I lie in bed in Michael's arms one night and tell him, "This is the first time in years that I am truly happy!"

. . . which is an idiotic and dangerous thing to say!

In Jewish folklore, declaring your good fortune aloud arouses envy and tempts the Evil Eye. To ward off this malicious spirit, the very moment after saying something so carelessly self-congratulatory, you must spit quickly three times through your middle and index finger—*Tuh! Tuh! Tuh!*

Evil Eye? I'm neither superstitious nor religious. My assimilated Jewish parents rejected their own orthodox upbringings and kosher homes. They raised me and my two sisters without Hebrew school or bat mitzvahs. We celebrated the major Jewish holidays, supplementing our repertory with Christmas presents, Easter egg hunts, and marshmallow peeps.

My mother was a sociology professor with a well-developed sense of logic. But she retained some vestigial Old Country beliefs—from her father's Russian side, her mother's rural Oklahoma side, and her grandparents' Latvian side of the family—which she synthesized into an eclectic array of rituals and phobias.

When Mom spilled salt, she threw it over her left shoulder for good luck. When there was an electrical storm, she made us sit in the middle of the room, out of reach of sinister and highly motivated lightning bolts. When she taught sociology at City University, she walked up ten flights rather than take the death-defying elevator ride. When we went to the beach, Mom parked our beach towels twenty feet above the high tide line, in case a shark decided to evolve on the spot into a predatory land animal.

But her most powerful protection against the Evil Eye was to make sure she was never happy for too long, a lesson she repeatedly demonstrated for me.

I am three years old. I'm sitting on the floor, watching Mommy dance in her friend's living room, just for fun, for the pure joy of dancing. Her friend plays gypsy dances on the piano. Mommy spins and leaps, sweaty, red-cheeked, and laughing. "I love dancing!" she shouts, mid-leap. Then she crashes her foot into the piano bench and breaks her big toe. No more dancing.

I'm twenty-two. I have just graduated from college. Mom is fifty-seven. To prove to her that I'm a grown-up, I treat her to lunch at a nice, cheap Indian restaurant in the East Village. Mom has finally recovered from breast cancer and a long depression, and has found the teaching job of her dreams. Over vegetable pakoras and mango chutney, Mom tells me, "This is the first time in years that I am truly happy!"

We both forget about the Evil Eye. Mom speaks freely of her happiness. She arouses the envy of the gloomy professor at the next table. She neglects to break a toe. She doesn't park our beach towels far enough from the sharks. She leaves the spilled salt on the table by the chutney. She forgets to spit three times.

Two weeks later Mom died suddenly from a cerebral hemorrhage, caused by a ruptured aneurism.

So I should have known, happy as I was in the spring of 1999, that I was in grave danger. That the Evil Eye was lurking in the shadows, waiting for the moment when I dropped my guard and admitted to Michael aloud, with childlike glee and momentary suspension of my adult disbelief, "This is the first time in years that I am truly happy!"

Tuh! Tuh! Tuh!

One day in early April, three weeks after Michael and I were engaged, three weeks before my New School graduation, I woke up with an upset stomach. The nausea didn't go away. New symptoms emerged each day. Insomnia, mood swings, sore breasts, low energy, an urgent need to urinate. When I missed a period, I called Robin, my gynecologist.

"We expected that. When I switched you to the lower dose of estrogen, I told you that your period would end."

"But I've been so tired . . ."

"Welcome to menopause."

". . . and sick to my stomach."

"See a gastroenterologist."

I'm infertile.

When I was thirty and married to Brad, we wanted to have a baby. My period stopped for a year. One doctor said I lost my period because I had recently lost weight. Another insisted I was in menopause at age thirty. A third doctor suspected my fallopian tubes were blocked and sent me for a procedure called a hysterosalpingogram, which hurt like hell and which revealed my deformed uterus—*Bicornuate,* Latin for two-horned or two-chambered.

The deformity was caused by exposure to DES, *diethylstilbestrol,* the synthetic estrogen my mother took to prevent miscarriage when she was pregnant with me. I found out about DES when I was in college and *Ms.* magazine broke the story with the terrifying headline, "DES, Cancer Time Bomb!" My mother, heavy with guilt, brought me to her gynecologist to find out what injury she may have unintentionally caused me by taking the drug routinely prescribed as the "pregnancy vitamin." Since then, I've had an annual colposcopy—a microscopic examination of my cervix for possible cancer.

Dr. Zagami, recently voted Best Fertility Doctor! by *New York* magazine, told me, "Your estrogen level is so low, the only way you could ever become pregnant is by immaculate conception. I'm putting you on ERT, estrogen replacement therapy, which I ordinarily prescribe to menopausal women twice your age. You could get pregnant with fertility drugs, but I strongly advise against it. As a DES daughter, your cervix is likely to dilate early in the pregnancy, resulting in premature birth. And with your small, deformed uterus, there's no way you could carry a baby past six months, so you should never attempt to get pregnant. But look at the bright side; you'll never have to use birth control again."

That night I wept for a long time. Brad sat quietly on the bed and held me when I was too exhausted to cry anymore. Our grief satisfied Patricia, our social worker at Spence-Chapin adoption agency. She had met many infertile couples who treated adoption as an insurance plan, while secretly hoping to have a *real* baby, so that they could be *real* parents. We passed the cathartic grief test, and she signed us up.

We waited two years for a birth mother to choose us. Zoe was nineteen years old and didn't realize she was pregnant till her sixth month, when it was too late for an abortion. She wanted to go back to college. It wasn't the right time in her life to be a mom. We were at Julia's birth, and held her moments after she was born. Though we knew Zoe didn't want to raise a baby, it seemed like superhuman generosity for her to give her newborn baby to us. We were infinitely grateful to her for choosing us.

Julia has heard this story often. It is part of our family folklore.

At my New School University graduation ceremony in May of 1999, I walked down the aisle of the ornate chapel of Riverside Church feeling sick, anxious, and old. Michael was in the audience, briefly in town between performing gigs. He was touring for most of April. Tomorrow he would leave for two weeks in El Paso to create an original theater piece with Mexican American high school students. He had so much energy. I had so little. What happened to my eternal youth? Ubiquitous happiness? Was this menopause or was I sick? Was this misery my insurance policy against the Evil Eye, or did the Evil Eye cause this misery?

Dr. Kay, the gastroenterologist, sent me for an abdominal

sonogram and a CAT scan. He diagnosed me with anemia and reflux, and prescribed drugs and a low-acid diet. I asked him if I had to avoid drinking wine on our August trip to Italy.

"Have plenty of wine, especially the local reds! I'd never forgive myself if you went to Tuscany and didn't drink wine."

In July's heat, I felt worse. "My hip joints are sore, my breasts hurt, there's a hard swelling in my abdomen, I'm depressed, I can't sleep."

Dr. Kay sent me to his wife, Dr. Jan Riley, a general practitioner. She sent me for a breast sonogram and a hip X-ray, both negative. "Ask your gynecologist to adjust your estrogen level," she suggested.

With my feet in stirrups, I asked Robin about my symptoms, while she performed an internal exam.

"Why is my abdomen swollen?"

"Middle-aged loss of muscle tone."

"But my stomach has never been so firm in my life."

"You're a middle-aged woman in early menopause, and your figure is changing."

"Why do I feel like I have to pee all the time?"

Her rubber-gloved fingers pressed on my cervix and the walls of my vagina. "You have a bladder disorder called cystocele. Atrophied bladder muscle, a common symptom of aging. You'll experience some leaking when you sneeze and walk. The only way to cure it is with surgery, but the risks are worse than the cure."

She removed her gloves and examined my breasts.

"Why are my breasts so sore?"

"You have hard ridges as a result of wearing underwire bras for so many years."

"I don't feel ridges."

"I do."

"What about my depression and insomnia?"

"Welcome to menopause!"

"Can you retest my hormone levels?"

"No. I'd have to take you off the hormones for several weeks to get an accurate test, and your estrogen is too low to do that. Increase your exercise, start a weight-loss diet, continue the hormones, and see me in a year."

I dieted and forced myself to jog three miles a day, adding abdominal crunches and weight lifting to my regime. "Middle-aged loss of muscle tone," I reminded myself, popping the button on my pants, then popping a Premarin—*pre-* for *pre*gnant, *mar-* for *mare*, a female horse. My daily dose of pregnant horse estrogen.

Scene 3

Wedding Plans

Michael and I set a wedding date of June 11, 2000, which gave us nearly a year to plan. In July, while Julia was in LA, we visited the short list of wedding sites in our low-budget range, though I wasn't exactly in the mood. After Robin's diagnosis, I had a recurrent fantasy of walking down the aisle at my wedding, having hot flashes and wearing Depends, Michael looking like a college kid, holding hands with his ancient bride.

The round-faced young woman who gave us the tour of the Victorian wedding factory in central New Jersey wore a pale peach polyester bridesmaid dress, which matched the drapes, her hair ribbons, and her blush. Michael bated her with his charming smile and intentionally dumb questions. Unaware of Michael's sarcasm, she rattled off at lightning speed her script of menu options for the tightly scheduled nuptials, the breakneck pace of her delivery mirroring the pace of the ceremonies—eight weddings each weekend, a feat accomplished by herding the guests at each wedding to a different room every half hour.

The rustic Bear Mountain Inn, nestled in a beautiful mountain valley, was briefly the top contender, but we ruled it out when we returned with dozens of other betrothed couples for the complimentary food tasting, a parade of unidentifiable, identical fried things, variations on a theme of "pigs in a blanket," introduced ceremoniously as *fromage en croute* and *saucisses feuilletées*.

We weighed the merits of a civil service at City Hall, and reconsidered getting married at all. In late July, we found a place we both loved—an affordable, big old house in the country, ninety minutes upstate, with a wonderful in-house caterer. We paid our deposit and took a break.

Scene 4

Italy

It was our first vacation as a family. Julia, who would celebrate her ninth birthday in Tuscany, was an adventurous and uncomplaining traveler—open to trying anything new—especially gelato, but even the cathedrals and museums at which most kids balk. Michael, also on his first trip to Europe, had an obsessive drive to see everything, and set a manic sightseeing pace. We sped around Venice for three days, riding gondolas and water taxis, taking in Renaissance sculptures and the Biennale exhibit of contemporary art, viewing the city itself as a work of art slowly being submerged in water—like Michael's beloved and vulnerable hometown of New Orleans. At first I was energized by Michael's and Julia's high velocity tourist style. But each day I found it harder to keep up with them.

Driving into Tuscany, Michael at the wheel, he took a wrong turn and we ended up in downtown Florence, stuck in traffic outside the city hospital. My hand on my hard belly, I had a fleeting fantasy of checking into the hospital. I would point to my Berlitz phrasebook at the Italian for "What's wrong with me, Doctor?" He would smile condescendingly, borrow my book, and point to the phrase "Welcome to menopause!" which he would announce loudly in two languages, to the amusement of his colleagues. The Florentine traffic jam ended, Michael found the narrow, unpaved road we were looking for, and we drove up the mountain to our rented Tuscan cottage.

Signora Francesca Gimaldi, our eighty-five-year-old landlady, whose leathered face was crosshatched with wrinkles, greeted us in Italian. She took a grandmotherly shine to Julia and promptly flagged down the rickety local bus, returning three hours later with two brown paper bags filled with fresh figs—one for her and one for Julia.

Michael and Julia drove down the mountain to Florence over the next few days, to visit the Uffizi Gallery and to explore the city, but I was too tired to join them, so I stayed at our cottage. Signora Gimaldi and I rested on the gray slate patio together, two old ladies quietly gazing at the parched yellow grass, olive trees, and vineyards, the vines tethered to wooden stakes to support the ripening bunches of small, green grapes. I followed Dr. Kay's orders, and drank lots of local red wine.

Rome was beautiful but too hot to breathe. While Michael and Julia explored ancient ruins, cathedrals, and gardens, I became the American expert on Italian park benches. A Roman policeman shook me awake from a nap at the Villa Borghese Gardens and ordered me to leave.

I was famished, but after a few bites I couldn't eat. My cheeks were sunken, my stomach was bloated. On the last night of our trip, unable to sleep, I ran my hand over my abdomen. The swelling was bigger than at the beginning of our vacation. I put Michael's hand on my belly.

"What do you think it is?" he whispered, half-awake.

"Either I'm pregnant or this is a tumor."

"You'll be okay," he said uncertainly, his hand tracing the hard curve.

Back in New York City on Labor Day, I bought an over-the-counter pregnancy test kit. "Negative," I told Michael.

"How does that make you feel?" he asked.

"Relieved. Disappointed. Scared."

"Me too." He hugged me, picked up his suitcase, and left for the airport. He would be performing in Chicago all week, and would return late on Friday night.

What I Know

1. I have a large, hard lump in my lower abdomen.
2. I'm not pregnant.
3. I am forty-four and in early menopause.
4. I have been infertile since the age of thirty.
5. I have a bladder disorder.
6. I have sore breasts, a result of wearing underwire bras.
7. I've felt sick since April.
8. I'm anemic.
9. I'm depressed.
10. I have been on hormone replacement therapy for fourteen years, which increases my risk of cancer.
11. I'm a DES daughter, which increases my risk of cancer.
12. My mother had breast cancer.
13. I'm sure the lump is cancer.

Scene 5

Rosh Hashanah

The Jewish calendar is a combined lunar/solar calendar. The months correspond to the moon's cycle, the year to the Earth's rotation around the sun. Because twelve lunar months is eleven days short of a solar year, a thirty-day Leap Month is added every few years to keep in sync with the seasons. Jewish holidays begin at sundown, and the first evening is called "Erev" or "eve of." In 1999 the Jewish New Year, Rosh Hashanah, begins at sundown on Friday, September 10, four days after Labor Day.

That afternoon I had a 1:30 appointment with Dr. Jan Riley. In the waiting room I thought about anything to get my mind off the frightening bulge in my abdomen. *My first faculty meeting at The New School at 4:00 today. Rosh Hashanah dinner tonight at Sue and Larry's. Julia has a play date with their daughter, Adria, after school. I'll pick up a bottle of wine after my faculty meeting. Tomorrow I take Julia to Rosh Hashanah children's service. Her choice. Funny how I grew up with minimal Jewish education, I only go to synagogue on Rosh Hashanah and Yom Kippur, but Julia has been the driving force for her own Jewish education; she asked for Hebrew lessons from the age of six and is committed to having a bat mitzvah. So foreign to me, but I take her to Hebrew school every Monday with her friend Sophie. I adore Sophie's mother—we're on the cusp of a genuine friendship. Damn it, I've been waiting for Dr. Riley for two hours. I can't be late for my meeting.*

"How long have you had this?" asked Dr. Riley, pressing her hand on my swollen belly.

"I noticed it a month ago. My gynecologist said it was loss of muscle tone."

"Did she do an internal exam?"

"Yes."

"I'm sending you to Lenox Hill Hospital for an emergency CAT scan."

"I have a meeting for a new job in twenty minutes. Can I do this tomorrow?"

"No. I think you have a large uterine or ovarian tumor. I can't let you go the weekend without having this seen. It's Friday. Radiology closes at four. I'll call them and tell them to stay open for you."

It surprised me that I was so terrified to hear I had a tumor. It's what I expected. Michael wouldn't be back from Chicago till midnight, and was unreachable by phone. I called Sue from the hospital and told her I'd be late to dinner.

"Can I to come to the hospital to be with you?" Sue offered. "I can get Larry to take care of the kids."

"No, I don't want to worry Julia. Thanks for offering. I'm okay."

* * *

"This will make your organs glow," said the nurse in the crowded Radiology waiting room, handing me a quart of a gluey, white, vile-tasting liquid. "When you finish drinking it, take a walk, and come back in an hour."

In the middle of Central Park, in the center of this frenetic city, Turtle Pond is an oasis. On this insanely beautiful day, the sun was just slipping behind the treetops. A redwing blackbird perched on a cattail. A white heron gracefully fished along the far shore. Five turtles, lined up on a log, stretched their necks toward the afternoon's last rays of sun, toward the impossibly blue sky. The pond was framed by weeping willows, the willows framed by the Manhattan skyline. This might be the last time I would see Central Park in late summer. This might be my last Rosh Hashanah. Would I live long enough to marry Michael? To help Julia grow up?

I walked back to Lenox Hill. I was the only one in the now shadowy waiting room, except for Jim, the young, black-haired radiologist, and his white-haired assistant, Jane, who were staying late just for me. The incandescent lamps had been turned off, leaving a bluish glow over the reception desk. They ushered me into a fluorescent-lit room and hooked me up to an IV, which made my mouth taste like aluminum, and dyed my glowing uterus and ovaries—and whatever hard and unwelcome mass was growing in them—purple.

Directed by Jane over a loudspeaker, I lay down on a metal tube, which transported me inside the human-sized white cylinder, a sterile and profoundly lonely place. I wished I'd asked Sue to come to the hospital with me. Between repeated immersions in the cylinder, I glimpsed Jim and Jane through the glass window. Their faces, which I tried to read for clues, looked troubled and confused. Jane apologized over the monitor. "The X-rays aren't clear. We'll have to run it again."

When they were done, I sat in the chilly waiting area and fell asleep.

"Mrs. Cohen. Mrs. Cohen." Jim was gently shaking my shoulder. "We did find something in you, Mrs. Cohen."

"You did?"

"We found a baby."

"What?"

"We found a baby."

"What?"

"We found a baby in you. Congratulations, Mrs. Cohen!"

Obviously, this is a dream. I argue with him in my dream.

"That's impossible."

"Well, yes, we're very surprised. Your medical records say you're in menopause, and we didn't expect to find a baby. It's not customary to diagnose a pregnancy with a CAT scan. Not recommended. Nevertheless, as I say, there is a baby in you."

"I don't believe you."

"We found a baby."

Maybe this is a semantic misunderstanding—a slapstick "Who's on first?" dialogue, with "baby" a proper name standing in for something else. I try to figure out the joke.

"What do you mean by 'baby'?"

"I think you'd better come to the ultrasound room and see for yourself."

I can tell it's a dream by the script. It has that hard-boiled, noir dialogue of movies and dreams: *"We found a baby in you, Mrs. Cohen!" "I don't believe you!" "You'd better come to the ultrasound room and see for yourself!"*

Since my identity is predicated on my infertility, the statement, "Mrs. Cohen, we found a baby in you," made no more sense than if he'd said, "Mrs. Cohen, we discovered that you're a man." Or, "Mrs. Cohen, we found out that you're black." Or, "Mrs. Cohen, the CAT scan revealed that you're a billionaire, or a dog, or a registered Republican, or a right-to-life lobbyist." However, I'm beginning to believe the radiologist, in that way you believe what a dream character tells you, no matter how lunatic it might be. In fact I'm beginning to warm up to this idea of being A Little Pregnant instead of having A Big Tumor. Given a choice between a few life-affirming embryonic cells and a lethal mass of cancer cells, I'll take the embryo!

I can tell it's a dream because, as so often happens in my dreams, I'm both inside and outside myself. It's another recurrent dream of mine. I wrote a solo play about this dream of me, on the ceiling, looking at me on the examining table, looking at me on the video screen. It always starts out this way, in my dreams and in my plays, but I never know what's going to show up on the video screen.

The radiologist slathers my belly with warm gel and moves the ultrasound device—kind of like a computer mouse—over the gooey surface, matched by a slurpy, *gloop, gloo-oo-oop* sound. The video screen is filled with shifting patterns of gray dots.

Maybe, in this dream, the video screen is a Rorschach test,

an opportunity for self-analysis. In a dream a baby represents the self—I took a course on Freudian and Jungian dream analysis at Princeton—I'm going to give birth to my self.

He stops moving the sonogram camera over my gloopy belly.

Out of the gray haze, there is now a baby on the screen. It has a baby's profile, rather pretty, with a button nose, parted lips, and an enormous forehead. A rhythmic flickering of light is its tiny heart, quick as a little bird's heartbeat—*ta-tinn-ta-tinn-ta-tinn-ta-tinn*. . . . A thick, coiled umbilical cord floats from its baby belly, a teeny penis peeks between his legs. The baby has two feet, five toes apiece, two hands, each with five fingers.

He is waving his right hand. There's a distant, high-pitched voice from inside my head, a fairy's voice. "Hello, Mommy. I'm here. I slipped under the radar. I hid from you, but now I'm here, and I'm waving at you. See me? See me, Mommy? See me waving my little hand? See my heart? My little heart beating so fast, *ta-tinn, ta-tinn, ta-tinn, ta-tinn, ta-tinn*? Now you see me? Ha! Ha! Ha!"

"I'm here with Alice Cohen. . . ."

Jim is on the phone with Dr. Riley, while Jane silently pats my hand and smiles her worried, lips-together smile. "No malignancy. No. She's pregnant. . . . Yes, that's what she told me. . . . She's in her third trimester. Twenty-six weeks. . . . Yes, the fetus is moving, heart rate is good. . . . Your patient appears to be in shock. . . . You need to talk to her."

I wrench my brain out of believing I'm in a dream so that I can give all my attention to believing I'm in shock. That's as much as I'm ready to believe. The radiologist hands me the receiver.

"Congratulations, Alice, this is great news!"

"Dr. Riley . . . I don't want to have a baby. I can't have a baby. Can I get an abortion?"

"No, it's too late for that. An abortion is not legal after twenty-four weeks. This is really very good news, Alice, but you're in shock right now. I thought you had a tumor, I was afraid you had cancer, I really did, or I never would have sent you for a CAT scan. But you don't have a tumor. You're healthy. The fetus is healthy. Call me Monday and I'll refer you to a high-risk obstetrician. Go home now. Take it easy this weekend. Drink lots of water. Oh, and stop taking the estrogen! Start taking prenatal vitamins."

"Do you want to know the sex of your baby?" the radiologist asks.

"Yes. No. Please don't tell me."

I know already, but I don't want him to tell me. Knowing it's a boy makes it worse, somehow. If I don't hear it from the doctor, maybe I will have been mistaken and it will be a girl, or this will still be a dream.

But I know it's a boy. And I've rejected my son on the first day I met him. "I don't want to have a baby. Can I get an abortion?" I said out loud in front of three doctors. And worse, before rejecting my son, I neglected him for six months. I starved him, and probably injured him, subjected him to drugs and CAT scans, purple dye, Italian red wine and caffeine and X-rays. And now I don't want him. What kind of a mother am I? A monster.

"Take the sonogram image home with you. Your first baby picture."

* * *

It was night when I left the hospital. With a picture of my unborn son hidden in my pocket, I cabbed to Sue's and assured her I was okay but that I had to talk to Michael before I could tell her the results of the CAT scan. Julia and Adria sat to my left, Julia eating Sue's elegant meal of veal stew and wild rice in her characteristically messy style, Adria with precociously grown-up manners. Julia, happy to be out late with her friend, didn't notice that I was too distracted to carry on a coherent conversation, that I couldn't eat a bite of dinner, that I kept grabbing her hand under the table, like a child afraid of the dark.

Michael got home at 1:00 a.m. "I'm exhausted. Can't this wait till morning?"

"No."

He put his suitcase down and sat on the sofa with me.

"I'm six months pregnant."

He looked at me funny, checking to see if I was making a joke. I handed him the sonogram picture. He studied the grainy image, taking a moment before identifying the profile, the nose, the parted lips, the feet and hands. He burst into tears. He was crying from happiness. I started crying. With Michael home, holding each other and crying, I think I was happy. That's what it was that night. Happiness.

Friday, terrifying and surreal, is over. I don't have cancer. Michael is with me. We're getting married. We're going to have a baby. Julia will have a little brother. We're a family. My son waved at me, his heart is beating, he has ten fingers and ten toes. To life! L'chaim! A sweet New Year!

ACT II

What I Know

Days of Awe

Rosh Hashanah. Saturday, September 11, 1999.

This is what I know:

1. I'm six months pregnant.
2. It's a boy.
3. It's too late for an abortion.
4. I'm not in menopause.
5. My cervix is likely to dilate at any time.
6. My uterus is small and deformed.
7. I can't carry a baby past six months.
8. A baby born at six months will probably die. If it survives it's likely to be severely disabled.
9. In six months of pregnancy, I've had no prenatal care, no weight gain, X-rays, CAT scans, lots of meds, lots of Italian red wine.
10. I took synthetic hormones every day of the pregnancy.
11. Synthetic estrogen causes birth defects. It caused my birth defects from DES.

12. Exhaustion, nausea, anemia, frequent need to uri-
    nate, sore breasts, sore hip joints, and reflux are all
    symptoms of pregnancy.

13. I didn't need to take estrogen.

14. I took prescription pregnant horse estrogen for
    fourteen years.

15. I was never infertile.

16. A home pregnancy test is only accurate in the first
    trimester.

17. Dylan was right when he told me in March that I
    was pregnant.

The Jewish High Holidays are called the Days of Awe. On the eve
of Rosh Hashanah, God opens the Book of Life and inscribes the
fate of every human being in it—who shall live and who shall
die, who shall be healthy and who sick, who shall be happy or
unhappy—but God's judgment is not finalized until the book
is closed ten days later, on Yom Kippur, the day of fasting and
atonement. "On Rosh Hashanah it is written, on Yom Kippur it
is sealed."

I did not take Julia to the Rosh Hashanah children's service,
as I'd planned. I had to find an obstetrician. Pregnancy trumped
synagogue. Michael and I told a few people about my pregnancy:
Julia. My sisters, Madeline and Jennifer. Michael's sister, Chris-
tie, and his mother, Daisy. My dad. Sue.

"Julia, sit down. We have exciting news," we told her on Saturday morning.

"What?"

"I'm going to have a baby."

Julia's eyes opened wide and her jaw dropped, like in the cartoons. "Really?"

"Really. In three months."

"Excuse me while I drop dead for a minute. Bleh!" She flopped over on the couch.

Michael and I laughed. Julia bounced back up.

"Could you tell me that again?"

"I'm going to have a baby in three months."

"Excuse me while I drop dead again. Bleh!" She flopped over again on the couch, bounced up again.

"Wait a minute. Didn't you tell me that a long time ago your doctor said that you could never have a baby, and that's why you adopted me?"

"The doctor made a mistake."

"Excuse me while I drop dead again. Bleh! . . . Wait a minute. Does that mean that this baby will be yours and Michael's baby? Will I be the sister? Or will I be the half sister? Or the stepsister? Wait a minute, what does that make me?"

Julia had for several years begged me for a baby sister or brother, but recently had dropped that request and appreciated her rock-solid status as a single child hugely outnumbered by parents and grandparents—me, Brad, Michael, her off-site birth parents (not an active presence, but part of her backstory), and Julia's gaggle of grandparents—my dad, Brad's parents, Michael's parents. It was now dawning on her that she might not be permanently assured her position as the center of our collective universe.

Untouchable

A pregnant woman with no prenatal care for twenty-six weeks is a lousy insurance risk. She might be a drug addict, an alcoholic, an illegal alien, a criminal, a teenager, crazy, deluded, HIV positive, uninsured, or—worst of all—litigious! To an obstetrician, she represents an expensive malpractice liability and higher insurance premiums. A forty-four-year-old pregnant woman in her third trimester, with a deformed uterus and no prenatal care can be, for an obstetrician, professional suicide.

No high-risk obstetrician would see me. I was an Untouchable. Sue recommended Dr. Carrie Rosenbloom, a celebrated high-risk ob-gyn who recently delivered twins for Sue's friend Erica. Rosenbloom spoke to me on the phone. It was against her policy to take on a new patient so far into a pregnancy.

My insurance plan, I discovered, sucked. I had Oxford's Liberty Plan (bad), not their Freedom Plan (not-so-bad). Liberty was the only Oxford policy that freelancers could buy. Doctors despised it because they were paid so little and so late.

"I called all the high-risk obstetricians I know," said Dr. Riley on Monday, "but no one will see you this far into the pregnancy. Ask your insurance company for a referral. I'm afraid there's nothing else I can do for you. It's outrageous that your gynecologist did an internal exam when you were five months pregnant. Just unbelievable! Have you spoken to her? I think you should call her. It's an outrage."

* * *

"Robin, I was five months pregnant when you examined me."

"You weren't five months pregnant!"

"You did an internal exam on me six weeks ago. And I just found out Friday—through an emergency CAT scan—that I'm six-and-a-half-months pregnant."

"Oh . . . Alice . . . I'm so sorry."

"I'd like a referral for a high-risk obstetrician," I said to the Oxford telephone agent.

"What is the nature of the risk?"

"There are several. I'm forty-four years old, I'm six months pregnant, and I've had no prenatal care."

"What is the pregnancy risk?"

"Um . . . advanced maternal age?"

"Just a moment, please. . . . That's not a risk factor."

"Yes, it is."

"There's no code number for it, so it's not considered a risk factor."

"That's ridiculous!"

"We don't have an age policy regarding high-risk ob-gyn treatment. You said there were other risk factors?"

"OK. I'm a DES daughter—Di-ethyl-stilbestrol. Because of my DES exposure in utero, my cervix is likely to dilate early, resulting in premature delivery."

"Just a moment, please. . . . There's no code number for DES."

"There's no code for DES, because DES daughters are too old to have babies!"

"Are there any other risk factors, Ms. Cohen?"

"Yes. I have a deformed uterus. That has to be on your list. A small, deformed, two-horned, bicornuate uterus."

"Could you spell that?"

"B-i-c-o-r-n-u-a-t-e."

"Just a moment, please. . . . There's no code for that."

"Please listen for a minute. I'm forty-four years old; I've had no prenatal care for six months; I've been given hormones that are dangerous for the fetus every day of the pregnancy; my cervix is likely to dilate early; I have a deformed uterus; and I've been told I can't carry a baby past six months, which was two weeks ago."

"According to our codes, none of these qualify you for high-risk obstetric care. Is there anything else I can help you with today, Ms. Cohen?"

My sister Madeline came to the rescue with a referral for her friend's high-risk ob-gyn. Dr. Slotkin agreed to see me, though he didn't accept Oxford, so I'd have to pay out-of-pocket.

"Yes, I'm very familiar with DES daughters. If I'd seen you earlier in your pregnancy, I would have put a stitch in your cervix to keep it from dilating, but it's too late for that. If I put a stitch in now, it would probably cause your cervix to dilate, and that's exactly what we don't want. I'd like you to take it easy, Alice, really limit your physical activity."

"Can we do an amnio?"

"Well . . . since it's too late for an abortion, amniocentesis is pointless, and there is a slight risk involved in the procedure. However, if there is a serious genetic defect—amnio only tests for a few genetic disorders: Down syndrome, cystic fibrosis, the big ones—it might be legal to have a late-term abortion."

I shocked myself by wishing for a serious genetic defect so that I could have an abortion and get on with my life. "I want to do amnio right away."

He hesitated, then told me a story. "My big brother has Down syndrome. My parents' lives were turned upside down by the relentless demands of raising Howard. He lives in a state institution now. I don't know if he's ever been happy, it's so hard to tell. . . . Given your advanced maternal age, Alice, you're at greatly increased risk of genetic defect. I understand why you want amnio, and why you would choose an abortion. I won't judge you, if this is how it plays out. But let's hope the baby is healthy."

It pinched when the doctor drew amniotic fluid from me. On the ultrasound screen I watched the sonographer enter measurements of the baby's limbs and head. He cheerfully pointed out the baby's penis on the screen, and produced an estimated due date.

Two days later Dr. Slotkin called with the test results.

"The fetus is genetically female but anatomically male."

"I don't understand."

"She has a double X chromosome and male anatomy."

". . . She's a girl with a penis?"

"Yes."

"Why? Why does . . . why does she have a penis?"

"I don't know. It's very unusual."

The shock of carrying a girl with a penis tricked me momentarily into thinking I was hearing difficult news about an ordinary pregnancy. Then I remembered how bizarre every aspect of this pregnancy was.

"Does this make it legal to get a late-term abortion?"

"No. It's not necessarily a health concern, so it doesn't meet the state requirements for late-term abortion. I would like you to see Dr. Katzen, a pediatric urologist surgeon who has experience with ambiguous genitalia."

The Surgeon

Dr. Katzen proudly turned the pages of his portfolio. "Here are twins Jerome and Joshua."

Photo of two baby boys, as macho as two infants in blue onesies can be.

"Turn the page. Jerome and Joshua are now . . . Jessica and Janice!"

In this photo, the babies are now in pink dresses, looking *très femme.*

Dr. Katzen looked across his desk to make sure Michael and I were suitably impressed. We nodded, speechless. Sketching on pink Post-it notes, he enthusiastically showed us how he could create a sexual metamorphosis with a scalpel and needle. He was a veritable Michelangelo of the pediatric operating table, a baby's genitals his virgin slab of marble. He could cosmetically sculpt our baby's two-inch penis into a compact little clitoris.

"Won't she lose sexual sensation?" I asked, my voice suddenly hoarse, a shudder running the length of my body. I grabbed

Michael's hand, which was cold and shaky. He didn't want to be here. He was here because I'd asked him to come. "Can't we just wait till our baby is born and see what happens?" he'd said, but I didn't think I could handle any more surprises.

On a blue Post-it, the surgeon drew a picture of the long nerve that runs the length of a penis. Then on a pink Post-it he drew that same two-and-a-half-inch nerve, neatly folded multiple times, to fit in her new, improved, half-inch clitoris. "By preserving the nerve, we are able to preserve sexual sensation and optimize adult sexual function."

"Wow, wow, wow!" I said, shuddering again, imagining how it must feel to have the nerve that transmits sexual sensation folded up and sewn into a teeny satchel, and I shuddered again when I imagined the doctor sneezing and missing just when he was adding the final trim.

Dr. Katzen sketched some more, on gender-neutral yellow Post-its, to show us how he could create a functional vagina in our baby, should hers be missing.

"Wow!" What else could I say to the surgeon who promised he could turn my baby's penis into a clitoris, and fabricate a vagina into my vagina-less little girl.

"Have you done many of these surgeries?" I ask.

"No. Just a few. As many as any surgeon has. Genital ambiguity is extremely rare."

"Is surgery always recommended?" Michael asked.

"The American Medical Association recommends corrective surgery for children with ambiguous genitalia." Katzen's face darkened. "However, the transgender activists are against it. They abhor the term *normalcy*. They say surgery robs them of their unique gender identity and diminishes sexual sensation. They think every child with ambiguous genitals should have the privilege of saying, 'It's my body, it's not like anybody else's body, and I like it the way it is.' Which is total bullshit! How is a twelve-year-old boy without a penis going to feel when the other boys taunt him in the locker room? How will a teenage girl with a penis feel when her boyfriend rejects her in disgust? It's cruel to subject boys and girls to that kind of humiliation!"

He cleared his throat and settled back in his chair. "I urge you to consider surgical correction."

Michael and I took his sketches home with us.

We've known for less than a week that we're having a baby in three months. Now we have to face the ethical dilemma of whether to surgically correct her penis. Katzen's solution sounds at least as dogmatic as that of the transgender activists, and terrifyingly irreversible. In the meantime, the gender ambiguity made choosing a name . . . complicated.

Salt-Wasting

Genital ambiguity has few known causes. Exposure to excessive hormones in utero, such as the synthetic estrogen I was taking for the first six months of pregnancy, can cause birth defects, including genital deformity. It can also be caused by CAH (Congenital Adrenal Hyperplasia), a rare, salt-wasting genetic disease, fatal if not treated daily. Genital ambiguity is the only outward physical sign of CAH.

Dr. Wong, at New York Hospital, was an expert on Congenital Adrenal Hyperplasia. Her beautiful young associate Dr. Melina Christopoulos wore a short white robe over her red miniskirt and thigh-high black boots. Her Greek-accented breathy voice enhanced her hot-chick-in-a-doctor's-robe look.

"All you need is love for baby," says Dr. Christopoulos. "Do not worry for CAH. Like diabetes, but easier. No shots. Give one pill a day, or she will die. So easy. All she needs is love and one pill. CAH girls are strong and athletic. Many grow up to be lesbians. But I think your baby does not have CAH. I think her penis is from estrogen pills Alice took during pregnancy. I will look at baby on day she is born. If genital ambiguity, I will take her to emergency room to rule out CAH."

"It's going to be okay, Alice," says Michael.

I don't share his confidence.

At home, I read the twelve-page patient information insert from my hormone prescription. *"Do not take during pregnancy. . . . Deformities in newborn rats when taken during pregnancy. . . . Abnormal masculinization of female genitals."* The pill I took every day for the first six months of pregnancy caused this baby girl to have a penis. And who knows what other injuries, as yet undetected, she has; what cancer time bomb might detonate?

"You're overthinking this," says Michael, accurately.

What have I done? Fourteen years ago I'd longed to get pregnant and have a baby. Fourteen years ago, I knew I would take care of my baby from the beginning of my pregnancy. I would never bring a baby into the world this way! I've injured her. Let me start over.

But *start over* is my not-so-secret code for *abortion*, and it's too late for an abortion, and this is too terrible a thought to tolerate now that we've all said yes to this baby and yes to being a family.

"She'll be our baby, she'll be great, we'll be great," says Michael, and he means it. But he can tell he's not getting through to me. He can tell I'm tumbling into an abyss, and it scares both of us.

I had been unhappy before, but I had never thought about killing myself. I've never been able to watch violent scenes in movies. I usually close my eyes before the shooting starts. Now when I close my eyes, and sometimes with my eyes open, I see violent scenes in which I play the central, fatal role.

What I Know

1. I'm having a baby girl in three months.
2. Unless she's premature.
3. She probably has a penis.
4. Genital surgery can change her penis into a clitoris.
5. Surgical correction is recommended by the AMA.
6. Surgical correction is considered unethical by people with genital ambiguity.
7. She may have a fatal disorder.
8. She will be a lesbian athlete.
9. I have uncontrollable thoughts about killing myself.
10. I have too many responsibilities to commit suicide.

Scene 2

Yom Kippur

"On Rosh Hashanah it is written. On Yom Kippur it is sealed."

Aware of my suicidal fantasies, Sue called her well-connected friend Erica, who called her well-connected aunt Charlotte (a chapter president of Planned Parenthood), who called her brother, Erica's father (a well-connected doctor), who pulled some strings for me to see Dr. Raushbaum, a feared and revered abortion specialist at New York Hospital.

I go to synagogue two times a year, on Rosh Hashanah and on Yom Kippur. This year I started Rosh Hashanah in the metal cylinder of a CAT scan. I would spend Yom Kippur, the Jewish day of fasting and atonement, in Dr. Raushbaum's office arranging for a late-term abortion. It was ten days after I found out I was pregnant.

Michael came with me. Seventyish and stout, the doctor sat in an old leather chair at a heavy wooden desk, heaped with unsteady mountains of papers. He chewed on an unlit cigar and inspected us over his beakish nose.

"Tell me exactly how it came about that you are six months pregnant but you didn't find out about it until last week."

I told him.

"Your story is remarkable. Your doctors are incompetent idiots." He leaned over his desk, rolled his cigar around with his tongue, and glared at me. "You're also an idiot! You were in denial for the past six months. Every woman knows subliminally when she's pregnant. You must have felt the baby kicking, didn't you?"

"No, I didn't."

He dismissed my protests with a snort, a wave of his hand, a roll of his cigar. "Let's get to the business at hand. Tell me why you requested this urgent meeting on Yom Kippur, the holiest day of the year, the day God decides who is and who is not inscribed into the Book of Life. Not that I care, I'm an atheist."

"I don't want to have a baby. I'm depressed and terrified. I had no prenatal care for the first six months, and the baby was subjected to drugs and X-rays, a CAT scan—"

"Yes, and?"

"—And she's a female but she has a penis, and she might have CAH, a fatal salt-wasting—"

"Yes, and?"

"—And I'm scared I'll go into labor any day and the baby will be premature and severely disabled and—"

"Yes, and?"

"Why do you keep saying, 'yes, and'?"

"Is your life in danger?"

"What do you mean?"

His thick eyebrows joined to form one thick line. "I don't

have time for stupidity. Why are you in my office? I can't legally put words into your mouth. Exactly how depressed are you?"

"I think about killing myself."

"Thank you! I'm sorry you're so unhappy, but that's why we're here, isn't it? Since you're contemplating suicide, the mother's life is in danger, which is the only way you can get a legal abortion. Not in New York State, which has no exception to the twenty-four-week limit. You could, however, have an abortion in Wichita, Kansas."

I can't think of a less likely place for liberal abortion laws. I've been to Wichita. My very first solo tour, when I was twenty-eight, was two weeks in south-central Kansas. Antigay and anti-abortion protesters accosted travelers in the airport with leaflets and recruitment entreaties.

"In Kansas, if the mother's life is in danger, an abortion is legal up until the twenty-eighth week. Seven days from today. Do you want me to call the abortion clinic in Wichita right now?"

I nodded. He called Wichita and scheduled an abortion for Tuesday, in one week.

"Now it's in your hands. You can call and discuss it with them. You can think about it for the next few days before you decide. Meanwhile, I'll get you an appointment with Dr. Carrie Rosenbloom. She is the only doctor you should be seeing for this pregnancy. The best high-risk obstetrician in the country.

"I already called her. She wouldn't see me."

"She'll see you, because I'll tell her to. And let's get the goddamn penis question straightened out. It's hard to read a sonogram. It's a bunch of gray dots on a screen. Your guy might have thought he saw a penis, but maybe he saw the umbilical cord, or some other gray specks. There's a guy here who's the best sonographer in the world. He's going to look at the baby. But he's Catholic and a right-to-lifer with eleven kids, so don't let him know you're considering an abortion."

"He would allow his religious beliefs to affect the way he reads a sonogram?"

"Of course he would. A doctor is a person. We see what we see through a variety of lenses—the lens of science, of politics, religion, our personal passions. Reading a sonogram is not an exact science. If you mention abortion, he'll view the ambiguous gray dots on the screen through his right-to-life lens, and I guarantee you he will not see a penis."

Raushbaum swiveled his chair toward Michael. "What do you think about all this?"

"Me? Oh, Jesus . . . a lot of different things. I've seen Alice in the throes of this terrible unhappiness and . . . I don't recognize her. And I think her . . . misery is actually less about having a baby than it is about losing her freedom to choose. She feels imprisoned, and it's . . . it's making her go crazy. So for the first time in my life—and I come from an extremely conservative, antiabortion, southern Christian family where the abortion issue is totally black and white, no room for discussion—I'm sick just imagining what my family would even think if they knew we were talking to you about—For the first time, I've had to genuinely think about abortion rights. It's always been an abstraction. I've been politically in favor of choice, but uncommitted on the personal side. Because it's suddenly so real and imminent a question in our lives, I . . . for the first time I understand the importance of a woman's right to choose. But the equally compelling personal truth for me is that there's a baby. Our baby. My baby. And I don't care if she has a penis or two penises or a salt-wasting disease or three heads or . . . I can't stand the thought of this baby being aborted. So if Alice has an abortion, I won't go to Wichita with her. And I might not be here when she gets back. I'll have my own unbearable sorrow about losing this baby, about endorsing this decision. I'll have that sorrow for the rest of my life. But I don't want Alice to kill herself. So she should do what she needs to do. That's what I think about all this."

Dr. Raushbaum nodded at Michael, leaned back in his leather chair, chewed on his cigar, and looked at me.

"I have a two-year-old grandson. He's cute, but I get bored of him after twenty minutes. It takes forever to raise a child till it's old enough to be interesting. I couldn't do it again. But I'm not you. I wonder what you'll decide."

"I don't see a penis! I see a large labia and a large clitoris!" shouts the evangelist sonographer from New York Hospital at the gray shapes on the monitor. He knows the referral has come from well-known abortion doctor Dr. Raushbaum, who considers him the best sonographer in the world.

"I see a small penis and partially fused scrotum," declares the sonographer in Boston, whom Dr. Rosenbloom considers the best sonographer in the world, to whom she has sent me for a third opinion.

*   *   *

Michael and I halfheartedly pretend the four-hour drive home from Boston is an ordinary outing. We don't talk about the contradictory, inconclusive readings we've gotten from the world's greatest sonographers. We don't talk about Wichita. We listen to the radio, switching to stations with the best reception as we drive south. I briefly get National Public Radio.

"In the next few weeks, somewhere in the world, a baby will be born. And that baby will bring the world population to six billion! The UN has prepared a report called 'The World at Six Billion' in response to the global attention to this historic milestone and widespread concerns about overpopula—" The rest of the story is obscured by static.

"I hope our baby isn't the six-billionth," I say, contemplating the terrible possibility of giving birth in the next few weeks, considering my options.

"Yeah, I'm with you." Michael sighs, surfing stations. He turns off the radio. We drive in silence for a while. I watch scenery fly by. The trees in Massachusetts are beginning to turn color.

"I'm performing at that conference in Cleveland this week."

"When do you leave?"

"Tomorrow morning."

"Tomorrow!"

"I know, the timing is terrible."

"Yeah."

I look out the window and mope. We drive a bunch of miles.

"Michael . . ."

"What?"

"You're going to have to do something besides touring."

"What are you talking about?"

"If we have a baby, you can't be on the road so much."

"That's how I earn a living."

"I know, but I get the feeling you expect me to stay home and take care of the baby full time while you keep touring. Is that what you're thinking?"

"Thinking? I'm not thinking. I'm reacting. I'm dealing with the fact that you're very pregnant and very confused about it. So I'm sorry I haven't been planning a career change in the last two weeks, I've had other things on my mind."

"I can't raise a baby alone, with you on tour all the time."

"What do you suggest I do instead?"

"I don't know. Something closer to home."

"Okay. No more touring, ever," he says in his most sarcastic voice.

We drive for miles in silence. The green blur of trees is punctuated with flashes of red.

"I'll just get an office job and sit in a chair until I die."

"—I'm not saying you have to get an office job."

"Of course you want me to get an office job. It'll be really good for our family. Hey, my father worked at an office job he hated for forty years, and then he died. No reason I can't do that too. It'll be great—"

"You don't have to get an office job."

"No, of course not. Because you know exactly what job would be right for me."

"Stop it."

I turn on the radio and surf channels. All I can find is a religious station.

"—President Clinton twice vetoed the bill, but Republicans on the Hill are preparing for a new fight and plan to reintroduce Partial Birth Abortion Ban legislation in Congress next month. Republican presidential candidate George W. Bush is proving himself a great friend to the Christian Right because of his outspoken support for the bill and his unwavering antiabortion—"

"Ugh." I turn off the radio. "I hope abortion isn't illegal by Tuesday, or it's the coat hanger for me," I say, in an attempt at gallows humor.

Michael doesn't say anything. I shouldn't have said anything about the abortion, certainly not a joke. We drive in silence. I imagine myself at home with a baby—a single mother in practice, if not marital status—Michael on the road, calling home now and then.

"You say you really want this baby. But you can't just say that and then go all over the country all the time."

"I'll never leave our apartment again."

"You want complete freedom to go wherever you want, whenever you want, and that's been great up till now. You don't want to grow up, it's who you are, I've always loved that about you. But it makes me wonder if you've really thought about what it means to be a father, and if you really want this, because you can't have complete freedom *and* take care of a baby."

Michael starts to speed up. "I'm trying to support my family!"

"I know that. If you could just find something that doesn't take you away from us so much of—"

"Like what? I have no idea what else to do!" His foot presses heavily on the pedal. "Tell me! Tell me! What? Obviously you know. Tell me what I have to do!"

"I don't know!"

Michael is driving really fast, aggressively passing cars on the highway.

"Pease slow down. We'll talk about this later."

"Later when? Later after Wichita or later before Wichita?"

"Tonight. As soon as we get home."

He's driving so fast, I'm scared we'll crash. I cover my face with my hands.

"Slow down!"

He does. We drive a bunch of miles in silence. Connecticut, the Constitution State, welcomes us with a blue highway sign. I turn on the radio and we listen to NPR for the rest of the drive.

Scene 3

The Wichita Option

The Wichita Women's Health Center telephone receptionist, with her friendly midwestern voice, explained the late-term abortion procedure. "Yes, ma'am, first they'll anesthetize the fetus so that it won't feel anything. You'll be sedated during this. Then the doctor will inject the fetus with a lethal drug—it will be painless to the fetus, ma'am. In order to make the delivery safer for you, the surgeon might sever the arms and legs of the fetus, of course after the lethal injection has taken effect. It's not a fast process, you have to be prepared for that, ma'am. It can take up to five days. Your cervix will be dilated over a one-to-four-day period. Then the doctor will induce labor, and the delivery will take place under sedation. . . . Yes, it's most likely that you will deliver a dismembered and stillborn fetus. . . . Yes, I know this is not easy to hear, Ms. Cohen. Then we dispose of the remains, unless you wish to make alternate arrangements. Some women choose cremation or burial.

"I do need to inform you, as well, ma'am, that there is antiabortion hostility directed at our center. There are protests outside the center every single day. We have had some violent incidents. I must advise you to make reservations at the one hotel in town that is safe and secure for our patients. You should reserve a room right away, while you are contemplating this decision. And there is only one taxi service in town that will be safe and secure to take from the hotel to the women's health center. You will stay in the center for two to five days and then stay at the hotel for another two days to recuperate. During that time, you can come into the center to be seen by our doctors and our counselors.

"We recommend that you have someone come with you, Ms. Cohen. It can be painful to go through alone—physically and emotionally. But if you don't have someone with you, our counselors on staff will be available to talk to you before and after the procedure. We accept virtually all insurance policies. . . . Yes, even the Oxford Liberty Plan. . . . You can change your mind, even the same day. We are here to serve the needs of our patients."

"I wonder what I would do if I were in your shoes," said Dr. Rosenbloom, while looking at the sonogram on the video screen. "You and I are the same age. I have no idea what I would do. By the way, I can see why you didn't feel any kicking. The placenta is positioned at the front of the uterus, so it cushions the baby's kicks. You probably thought you had gas."

She told me to cancel all of my performances and avoid any physical exertion and to let her know of my decision.

* * *

"You'll do whatever you want to do. Let me know what you decide," says Michael, assaulting his suitcase with neatly folded business suits, costumes, and props. "If you abort this baby, I guess I'll move somewhere in the middle of the country and work at a 7-Eleven or something." He picks up his bags and leaves for the airport for a week in Cleveland.

My sisters Madeline and Jennifer stay close by me for the next few days. They don't want me to make this decision alone. They both advise me not to have an abortion. They won't go with me to Wichita, for practical reasons, they say—too short notice, busy at work—but they're protesting this abortion. Madeline and Jennifer are both staunch advocates of abortion rights, and I'm surprised not to have their support.

"You're too far into the pregnancy now," said Madeline.

"Michael will be such a great father," said Jennifer.

"I hope you have the baby. I have a feeling everything will work out," said Madeline.

I don't want to lose Michael.

I don't want to have a baby.

But my baby has already waved at me, so I guess she thinks it's a deal.

"You're such a mommy," said Jennifer. "You love children so much. Think about how much you love Julia. If you abort this baby, for the rest of your life you won't know if you did the right thing."

And if I don't abort this baby, for the rest of my life, I won't know if I did the right thing.

It's Monday, the last day of summer. I've booked a flight to Wichita tomorrow. I would have to go out alone. I am terrified of the physical procedure. I'm afraid of the angry mob of Kansans. I'm scared of what will happen to me physically, psychologically. I'm terrified of being in Wichita by myself for this horrific ordeal. I'm terrified of what will happen physically, the dismembering and—the killing of the fetus. The killing. The killing of what might be a viable baby. Not knowing for the rest of my life if I did the right thing.

I cancel my flight to Wichita and my appointment at the Women's Health Center.

I hang up.

My mind is racing, projecting a rapid-fire slide show of everything that's happened in the last six months. I start to hyperventilate, try to calm myself.

I close my eyes and talk myself into breathing slowly.

I lift my shirt and run my hands over my belly, the skin stretched tight over the newly globe-shaped center of my life, which rises and falls with each long inhale and exhale. Then something new. A small tremor, directly under my right hand and also deep inside. It's subtle. . . . Another. . . . I feel the baby kicking.

The phone rings. It's Michael in Cleveland.

"Please don't go to Wichita."

"I've already decided not to go."

"Thank God!"

He cries for a while. Then we're both quiet. Then he says, "Last night, my friend Beverly said, 'There's a reason God makes human gestation take nine months. It takes that long to get used to the idea of having a baby. You guys missed out on the first six months.'"

"Yeah, we did."

"We'll catch up."

"I hope so."

"I love you. I have to go. I perform in ten minutes."

I'm having a baby.

I don't know what will happen after that.

I buy three pairs of maternity pants, with elastic stomach panels.

The next morning I walked Julia to school. It was the second week of school. None of the other parents, many of whom were friends, knew I was pregnant. Even at six and a half months I was barely showing, so nobody asked.

Julia's school was only two blocks from our apartment. As we crossed Broadway, holding hands, I had a contraction and was doubled over in pain in the middle of the street. I made it to the median and told Julia I would watch her walk to school from there. She nodded seriously, carefully looked both ways, and crossed the street. It was the first time Julia had ever crossed a street by herself. When she reached the sidewalk, she turned around and waved, looking for encouragement. I waved back and blew her a kiss. She ran down the long block and I held my breath as she waited for the crossing guard to help her cross Amsterdam Avenue, even more treacherous than Broadway, a thunderous river of trucks and cabs.

Scene 4

My Left Side

Dr. Rosenbloom prescribed bed rest for the duration of the pregnancy. "Drink at least two quarts of Gatorade a day. Keep hydrated to prevent contractions. No sex. Only get out of bed to go to the bathroom, have a meal, or go to an appointment that is essential for your health."

"What about editing my theater journal? I can't afford to lose this job."

"Edit it in bed on your left side."

"What about teaching my college course on Monday nights?"

"Only if it's essential for your health."

"It's essential for my mental health."

"Then cab to and from your class. Take elevators, not stairs. Sit the whole time. Line up a sub and tell your class you probably won't complete the semester.

"Another thing, Alice. You know I don't accept your insurance plan. I'd like to keep you as a patient, but I understand if you prefer to see a doctor in-network. I can try to find somebody good for you. But frankly, I don't know anybody who accepts Oxford Liberty."

"I don't want to change doctors."

I canceled all my performances through the end of the year. Canceling twenty-five public library performances in South Jersey wasn't too painful, except for the lost income, which was alarming. The call to the Tampa Bay Performing Arts Center was really hard. I'd loved performing at TBPAC three years earlier, and the theater had contracted me to perform my new solo play in their experimental theater, and one of my family shows on the main stage.

Having divested most of my responsibilities and ambitions in the world outside of my apartment, I lay down in bed on my left side.

It was a relief to lie down, to give myself over to sleep. I had been feeling sick for six months. Now that my exhaustion was validated, I lay in a stupor, in and out of sleep. I wanted to be unconscious until the pregnancy was over, but my sleep was fractured and incomplete.

It was not a good bed, not a real bed, more of an improvised sleeping arrangement you might find in a college dorm. Michael's queen-size futon from his college life lay on a large sheet of plywood, supported by twelve of the wooden milk crates Brad found on the street twenty years before, when he was a penniless Juilliard student and his apartment was furnished entirely with milk crates. The futon was hard, and my left arm and leg kept falling asleep. Sue's friend Erica gave me the body-length pregnancy pillow she'd used when she was pregnant with twins. It helped. I draped my finally huge belly, my right leg and right arm over the body pillow, and dozed and woke and drank Gatorade and dozed and woke.

When I woke, I thought about this baby who would be disabled by prematurity, and by all the terrible things it had been subjected to for six months. I wished I could end the pregnancy, to save her. Killing myself would be one way of aborting the baby. It might be the most humane thing.

But I had too many responsibilities. I couldn't get the December issue of *Play by Play* out on time if I killed myself.

I couldn't kill myself because I needed and wanted to be there for Julia, whom I loved, whom I had always loved, since two months before she was born, when Zoe chose us.

I couldn't kill myself because I was in love with Michael, and, remarkably, he was still in love with me.

I couldn't kill myself because I had to take care of this baby inside me. I felt less like its mother than its intensive care unit. A barely mobile ICU, lying on its left side, to be loaded into a taxi and delivered to a hospital when baby was ready to be born. Thinking of myself as an ICU gave me a sense of purpose, a reason not to kill myself.

When I woke from my fitful naps, I attended to the slim remains of my freelance work. It took longer to write and edit my theater publication while lying in bed on my left side, drifting in and out of sleep.

I called my supervisor, a friend and colleague of many years, told her in confidence about my pregnancy and made a request. "I don't have access to an adequate insurance plan, and the baby might have special needs. Since I've worked for the organization for five years, do you think management might consider putting me on payroll, as an employee with benefits?"

"Gosh, Alice, this is just the wrong time to ask. The climate is all about belt-tightening, and benefits are a huge expense. I'm sorry, I just know what's up with management right now."

Julia missed me. She wished I could walk her to school and pick her up from school like I used to, but she was acting cheerful for me. She had her own key now. My friend Janet, mother of Julia's best friend, Emily, took Julia to and from school on days when Michael was out of town. Julia ran upstairs by herself, unlocked the door, climbed in bed under the covers with me, woke me with a kiss on my cheek, and told me about her day. Then she ran to the kitchen, ate a snack, and climbed back under the covers with me to do her homework.

This was my favorite time of the day. I loved having Julia close to me. She finished her homework under my covers, and got up to eat another snack. She was eating a lot these days. I thought she might be depressed, but I was so depressed I was sure I'd make her feel worse if I asked her about it. When he was in town, Michael made dinner—quesadillas, mac and cheese, pasta—and they ate in the kitchen together while I lay in bed listening to their conversations.

Michael was patient, nurturing, and consistent. He shopped for food. He cooked. When he wasn't touring his shows, he woke up in time to make Julia breakfast and walk her to school. He helped Julia with her homework. He went to the parent-teacher conference and the fourth-grade publishing party. He took her to Hebrew lessons. He coached her soccer team and spent most Saturday mornings with the West Side Soccer League. He listened patiently to my vacillating feelings of hope and hopelessness.

Michael behaved like a total grown-up. Like a saint. Fucking perfect. Who the hell was this guy? I didn't recognize him. I missed *real* Michael. Michael the trickster. The irrepressible, irresponsible, overgrown college kid who disappeared to play guitar and write songs and sleep crazy hours, and came back out of his cave when he was ready to be in a family again, when he was ready to make love again. Michael didn't have time to be himself. He was too busy taking care of me and Julia. He and I had both lost our selves to this pregnancy.

I was humiliated by being an invalid. Humiliated by Michael's ability to love this unborn baby when I could not. Overwhelmed by his generosity. Indebted to him. Jealous of his not having to lie in bed on his left side drinking Gatorade, which I found detestable no matter what flavor or color Julia picked out for me. I resented him for changing into someone else, someone who was unrecognizably patient and perfect and reliable and predictable and selfless and mature. Envied him for wanting this baby so instantly and completely. And of course I despised myself even more for having these contemptible feelings.

Three weeks ago I found out that I am pregnant.

Two weeks ago, I contemplated and rejected a late-term abortion.

One week ago I was put on bed rest.

I accepted my role as a miniature hospital, protecting a fragile life by lying on my left side and drinking Gatorade.

I told a few more people that I was pregnant. Congratulations from everyone I spoke to. Even when I judiciously divulged—to close acquaintances, to women I thought of as feminists—that I was unhappy, that this was terrifying, they laughed and teased and congratulated me again. "Lucky you! You thought you were infertile all these years, and you just had to find the right guy, and you didn't even have to take fertility drugs."

I could talk to my sisters and a few close friends who neither judged nor congratulated me.

Michael bought me a book of 1,500 baby names from Barnes and Noble. I read it and asked him to get me another book. "Isn't there one name in fifteen hundred you like?" He got me a baby name book with 2,739 names. This was great reading for an expectant mother who has to lie in bed all day. It had stories and history and etymology for every name. Each name conjured up a different child for me, so I got this idea that I could determine who this kid would be by naming her. Julia and I looked through the name book together under the covers after school. We only considered girls' names. With or without a penis, this baby was a girl. We made a list. Kate, Miranda, Anna, Louise, Helena . . . and Eliana, a Hebrew name. "Eliana's a pretty name," said Julia.

The translation of Eliana was "My God has answered me."

I wondered who Eliana might be, what question or prayer was answered.

I had way too much time, lying on my left side, to think, and I thought about this name and this baby.

Scene 5

Under the Radar

Eliana.

She wants to be born. She doesn't know she wants it. Against all odds, she is determined. And so she slips under the radar. She makes it into the Book of Life, just in time. Just as God is closing the Book at the end of Yom Kippur, she glides unseen between the covers and onto the page where her mother's and father's and sister's fates are also inscribed.

This is the reason for the name Eliana. "My God has answered me," the Hebrew translation. But from whose point of view? Whose God? Which "me"?

I think it's the baby's point of view, the baby's question, the baby's God. This baby wanted so much to be born that she slipped under the radar. Hid until it was too late to turn back, until she was ensured safe passage.

But it's generally assumed that it's *my* God who answered *me*, the fulfillment of my dream of fertility. The universal quest of barren, fairy-tale couples.

"The fisherman and his wife had long prayed for a child."

"The old couple, well past childbearing years, found a beautiful little girl in the open petals of a rose.

". . . in a seashell on the beach;

". . . in a basket on the doorway;

". . . the Old Farmer's Wife had always longed for a child. She drank the milk from a magic coconut and gave birth to a frog, and raised him as though he were a regular little boy."

"The barren witch stole baby Rapunzel and raised her in a tower."

"Lonely old Rumpelstiltskin demanded the first-born baby in exchange for weaving straw into gold."

What woman does not yearn for fertility?

"Congratulations!" is the only proper greeting to the pregnant woman, whatever her age or circumstances, but especially if she had been considered infertile, and her pregnancy is considered a miracle.

"Congratulations! When are you due?"

And if she's older, "Congratulations!" can be accompanied by laughter and teasing, with sexual innuendo.

"God said to Abraham, 'As for Sarah your wife, I will give you a son by her.'. . . Then Abraham fell on his face and laughed, and said to himself, 'Can a child be born to a man who is a hundred years old? Can Sarah, who is ninety years old, bear a child? GetOutaHere, Lord! My old wife?' said Abraham, rolling on the ground in paroxysms of laughter."

Or was God answering me?

This might have been the answer to my question at age thirty, when I longed for a child. If so, God is fourteen years late. Past the statute of limitations.

* * *

Tell me, Baby, was God answering you?

"Yes, Mama. I, miniscule trickster, pulled this one off, without benefit of consciousness, without benefit of breath or brain or lungs, with only the shadowy precursor of a beating heart. My first game of hide-and-seek. I hid for six months in the smaller horn of your two-horned uterus, staying as small and quiet and tucked in as I could, and tricked you into thinking I wasn't there. Every time you looked for me, I flipped to the other side of your womb, fooled you into not looking for me anymore, and then showed up unannounced on a TV screen—BOO!—Trick or treat, trick or treat! Give me something good to eat!

I'm a Hermaphrodite trickster,

Between and betwixter!

I'm waving at you, Mama.

I am Eliana! Eliana!"

I don't remember wishing for a baby. My wishes of recent years have more to do with slowing down, simplifying, streamlining, relaxing the demands of parenting, lowering the wattage on the challenges of survival, and returning to my creative work, now that my adopted daughter is finally big and strong and happy.

I try every day to want a baby.

* * *

At age forty-five, 75 percent of pregnancies end in spontaneous miscarriages. I reread the twelve pages of small print in the
ERT prescription patient information insert. *"Not for use during pregnancy. . . ."* The abnormally high level of estrogen might
have relaxed the muscles of my uterus, preventing the contractions that would likely have ended the pregnancy in miscarriage.
This miracle pregnancy may be the result not of prayer, but of
chemicals—the pregnant horse estrogen in my uterus. Nay!
Neigh!

Riddles

I call my father to tell him I'm pregnant.

"Congratulations! You'll finally know what it's like to be a
mother."

"I'm already a mother!"

"You know what I mean. Julia's adopted. Now you'll be a real
mother."

I miss my own mother.

When is a mother not a real mother?

What makes a mother real?

Biology?

Unconditional love?

Can a real mother's love be conditional?

Is she a real mother . . . if she doesn't yet feel love, hopes it will
awaken in her, and in the meantime gives up everything to protect the child?

Is she a real mother . . . if she thinks of her body as a mobile hospital, her womb an incubator, her pregnancy as the nursing task to which she devotes herself to protect this small life inside her, until its lungs are formed and its heart is strong?

Is she a real mother if she does exactly what she's told to do?
If she doesn't kill herself?
Is she a real mother if she is terrified at every waking and sleeping moment for the safety of the child?
Is she a real mother if she will sacrifice her life for the child inside her?

Is she a real mother if she said, out loud, when she first saw it on the video monitor, that she didn't want it?

Is a mother who contemplated aborting her six-month fetus a real mother?

What prevents a mother from loving?
When a woman is forced to be a mother.
When being pregnant makes her feel imprisoned and insane.

What is an infertile woman who has a baby?

Why did the baby leave the womb?
    To get to the other side?
    Because of the Hormones?
    Because she is a Miracle Baby?
    All of the above.

When is a baby a miracle?
When is a baby not a miracle?
Aren't all babies miracles?
What is a mother who loves all children except her own?
Is she still herself if she doesn't recognize herself?

Aunt Phyllis

I called my Aunt Phyllis.

"Alice, dahling, listen to me. You're being too hard on your-self. When I was pregnant with your cousin Walter in 1949, my obstetrician said—I'll never forget this!—he said, 'Phyllis, I like to deliver a small baby, a six-pound baby. I don't want you to gain more than twenty-five pounds.' So he put me on a diet, and I called him and said, 'But Doctor, I get so hungry,' and he said, 'Phyllis. If you get hungry, eat a candy bar.' And I called him again, and I said, 'But Doctor, I'm still hungry after the candy bar,' and he said, 'Phyllis. If you're still hungry after the candy bar, have a cigarette.' So I followed his instructions, and I smoked cigarettes all through my pregnancy. Do you think Wal-ter suffered? He's nearly six feet tall and he's the dean of the graduate school at Cornell University. So stop worrying."

Solo Theater

On the last Monday night of September, I get out of bed unsteadily, get dressed, and cab downtown to teach my solo theater class.

My class is enrolled to capacity. Fifteen students. New School University undergraduates and graduate students along with adult education students. A sixteenth student waits outside the classroom door and pleads with me to let her enroll. She's white-haired, blue-eyed, stout, seventyish, with folds of pale white skin. Under the wrinkles, her round face is like a little girl's, as is her fluttery body language, and the way she repeatedly pushes wisps of white hair from her eyes. "I drove here from Philadelphia and they told me your class is full, but I *have* to take this class. My name is Bella. They said at registration that you might let me stay." I invite her into the class. Sixteen students, ranging in age from twenty to seventy, look at me with great expectation. All these people desperate to create solo theater. Who knew? It was disorienting to sit upright, act like a normal person, interact with students, teach a class.

"All theater is storytelling," I tell my class, "but solo theater is a more primal form—akin to the ancient teller of tales, the Homeric bard, the African griot, the trickster, and the shaman. In this course we'll define 'story' and 'storytelling' very broadly. Other peoples' stories, your own stories, fantastical stories, stories with or without words. My goal is for each of you to find the story you want to tell and the way you need to tell it. The story you are compelled to tell right now might be different from the story you will want to tell a year from now. The way you tell your story now—the lens through which you view the story, the medium with which you communicate that story, the audience you want to reach—might be different from the way you tell that same story at another time in your life."

My students tell the class what brought them to a course in solo theater.

Jeremiah, a black poet from Alabama, handsome, with dreadlocks and glasses, is a year out of the military, getting his college degree, seizing a new life.

Dani Athena, pale and thin, with black hair and eyes—a choreographer, my age, who teaches dance at a high school, wants to finish a solo piece she started a few years ago.

Kayla, a nineteen-year-old African American girl from the housing projects in Red Hook, Brooklyn, has harrowing, half-finished stories to tell.

Bella, a librarian from Philadelphia, tells incoherent fragments with great urgency.

Richard, the prosecutor, tells stories for a living—"When I try a case, I tell a story with witnesses. The adversary tells a different story of the same set of events. My stories have to be disciplined, terse, and to the point. I want to learn to tell stories in a more narrative form."

Miriam wants to create a piece about her two dead grandmothers, still feuding in heaven.

I tell them I'm expecting a baby at the end of the semester, that I'm on bed rest but my obstetrician has allowed me to teach because this class was so important to me.

The idea of a fragile life inside of me, the fact that I'm taking a risk by teaching, sets the tone. It's a high-risk class. They treat the study of solo theater as if their lives depended on it, and as if my life depends on it, which it does.

For two hours a week, on Monday nights, teaching solo theater, cultivating this crop of storyteller-performers, I recognize myself again.

Adoption Option

I can give up the baby for adoption! Why didn't I think of this before? The symmetry is redemptive. When Brad and I were unable to have a baby, we received the gift of a child from Julia's birth mother, Zoe, who, like me, didn't know she was pregnant for six months. I will reciprocate and give this baby to a childless couple. Unlike abortion, this solution is morally unassailable. I am adoption's greatest advocate and happiest recipient. Julia is the poster child for adopted children. I'm adoption's poster mom.

"The baby doesn't need adoptive parents," says Michael. "She already has parents!"

Undeterred, I call Spence-Chapin adoption agency. "This is very ironic," I begin. "I adopted a baby through Spence-Chapin nine years ago. Now I'm pregnant and might want to give my baby up for adoption."

Eleven years earlier, when Brad and I first walked into the century-old mansion on Fifth Avenue and Ninety-fourth Street, we were given the historical tour. The side door was originally the entrance for pregnant women and girls, hidden from view to protect them from public shame. The grand front entrance was for the adoptive parents. These days, everybody—birth mothers and adoptive parents—enters through the front door; the side door is used for UPS deliveries.

Because I am on bed rest, Sasha the social worker comes to our apartment and gives us the lay of the land. "There are open adoptions, where the birth mother maintains a relationship with the child and the adopting parents. And closed adoptions, which are confidential, with no continuing relationship between birth mother and child. If the baby is healthy, there will be many potential adoptive parents. If the baby is sick or has significant special needs, there is a much smaller pool of potential adoptive families. Many of the parents who adopt special needs children are devout Christians who dedicate their lives to raising sick and disabled children in group homes.

"Since you haven't yet decided whether you want to give up the baby, right after the baby is born, we can arrange to have it placed with foster parents for up to a month while you decide."

Michael sits in on the session. "I'm trying to keep this family together," is all he says.

Sasha looks at Michael. "Legally . . ." she says, then pauses and looks at me. "Legally, the biological father has to give his approval before a baby can be placed with an adoptive family."

Michael looks at me, actively *not* giving his approval.

I think adoption is the right path. Michael disagrees, but our relationship is changing so rapidly, I can't predict what will happen. I persevere.

My sisters think this is a nutty idea. So do my friends. In this liberal, Upper West Side community, where abortion is accepted as a woman's inalienable right, giving up a baby for adoption is inconceivable. There are many adopted children at Julia's school, from all over the world, but it's a one-way option, ethically. Adopted children are accepted and valued, their parents perceived as heroic. Where I live, I'd be more harshly judged for giving up my baby for adoption than for having an abortion.

As an adoptive mother I want to fight for the moral defensibility of giving a child up for adoption. I want to start by correcting the distorted and misleading language of adoption. *Giving up a baby* sounds like abandoning it, throwing it away. But it's a gift. I want to *give*, not *give up* this baby, to a childless couple who will welcome her with the unambivalent devotion that eludes me.

"That's euphemistic and self-serving," says Michael.

"How can you say that when Julia's adopted?"

But what would it mean to Julia, as an adopted child, if her mother gave up her little sister for adoption. Would it open up an early wound, make her fear that I might give her away to someone else? And Michael, who is ready to be this baby's father, has never given me away or given me up while I've been on bed rest, hasn't rejected me while I've been not-so-quietly losing my mind, has been patiently and lovingly taking care of Julia, proving what a remarkable stepfather he is to her and what a wonderful father he would be to this baby.

Michael brings me a bottle of emerald green Gatorade. He sits on the edge of the bed while I prop myself on my elbow to take a few swigs.

"My mother says *she'll* adopt the baby," says Michael.

"That won't work."

"Obviously."

"I can't believe you told her we were considering adoption."

"*We* aren't considering it. *You* are."

"What else did your mother say?"

"She told me to be patient. She's says your emotions are out of whack because of your pregnancy hormones, and you'll snap out of it."

I have to get the fall issue of *Play by Play* to the printer. It's not easy editing from my futon office, left cheek mashed into my pillow, facing the telephone and laptop on Michael's side of the bed. The screen is perpendicular to my line of vision, so I prop it on Michael's pillow at a forty-five-degree angle and hope my left arm doesn't fall asleep before I finish typing. I'm having trouble maintaining my sense of professionalism.

Now my star student writer has stood me up, damn it! Yolanda is a twelfth-grader at a high school in the South Bronx. An articulate seventeen-year-old from the Dominican Republic, she's already been guaranteed a journalism scholarship and wants to study at Emory College. I've left a whole page blank for her review of a new play at Repertorio Español, which she has agreed to write in both Spanish and English, but she's missed her deadline and hasn't responded to my multiple e-mails or phone calls.

I leave another message on Yolanda's cell phone, trying to strike the right balance between supportive and scolding, between professional editor and maternal nudge.

"Yolanda. Please call me. Your extemporaneous review of the play on the phone last week was word-perfect. All you have to do is write it down."

Her call wakes me from a nap. "I'm really sorry to let you down, Ms. Cohen."

"It's okay, as long as you e-mail your review by—"

"I can't write the article."

"Then just make it up now, on the phone, and I'll type it for you."

"I can't."

"Why?"

Yolanda sighs deeply, almost a groan. "I just found out I'm pregnant. There's a lot to think about. I have to figure out what to do."

"Me too!" shouts my thought bubble. But I'm the grown-up here, Yolanda's mentor.

"I can imagine how difficult this must be for you," I say, trying to disentangle my numb left arm from the intertwined phone and power cords. "Do you want to talk about it?"

"I guess so. This is so confusing, cause my life was on a track that made me really happy, and this totally derails me. I mean, my boyfriend wants me to have the baby, but I want to be a journalist, right? I don't want to give up this scholarship. Nobody in my family has ever gone to college. If I have the baby I probably won't finish high school, so don't even talk about college. I feel like my future has just died."

I feel an intense identification with this seventeen-year-old grieving for her lost future.

"Do your parents know you're pregnant?"

"Are you kidding? My mom, she's Dominican—maybe you can't appreciate what that means—she's like having a party over this baby. She's knitting booties and mittens already, you know?"

"She's happy that you're pregnant?"

"Oh my God, totally! From the time I was fifteen she was like, 'Yolanda, chica, when you going to give me grandchildren?'"

"Wow. But what about your college plans?"

"Are you kidding? She doesn't want me to go to college! Emory College is in frickin' Georgia! She'll do anything to keep me home. She and my boyfriend are—they're like conspirators. I think they planned this pregnancy for me, to keep me home. Don't get me wrong. I'm equally responsible as my boyfriend, he didn't force me into anything. We used a condom, but it broke."

I feel the baby kicking and put my hand on my belly. Yolanda is the only other pregnant woman I've talked to since finding out that I'm pregnant—but she's not a woman, she's a girl. It's hard not to blurt out my story.

"You must think I'm an idiot, right? A stupid, pregnant teenager."

Which makes me what?—A pregnant, old idiot.

"I think you're a very smart and talented girl, with difficult decisions to make."

"I'm sorry I screwed up your magazine."

"You didn't screw it up, don't worry about it. Good luck with everything."

I wonder what Yolanda will decide, knowing I'll never hear from her again.

The fall issue of *Play by Play* is printed in a larger-than-usual font, with lots of photos.

* * *

It's late October. I haven't seen fall foliage. On my way back
home from my East Side appointment with Dr. Rosenbloom one
late afternoon, I ask the cabdriver to take Central Park Drive
and circle the park so I can see the fall leaves. He laughs and
warns me it will double the cost of the trip. There are some red
and gold leaves, but most are brown and many have fallen. Out-
doors, the season passes quickly, while in my bedroom, lying on
my left side, time is interminable.

Lamaze: First Lesson

Joy, the birth coach from New York Hospital, makes home visits. She comes Tuesday nights to tutor me and Michael in Lamaze
technique and give us tips on preparing for childbirth. She sets up
a flip chart in the living room. We sit on the sofa and watch the
show. Joy's a very funny lady who moonlights as a stand-up comic.

"One of my patients recently asked me, 'Is it okay to have
children after forty?' And I said, 'No, I think forty children is
quite enough.' *Ba-Dum Ching!* So where are you guys from?" Joy
shows us how to breathe, gives me some relaxation techniques,
and shows Michael how to massage me. He practices his massage technique later, in bed. Nice.

Adoption Visit

On Sasha the social worker's second visit, she brings a photo
album of hopeful adoptive couples, which she leaves with us.

"Look this over. When I come back next week, tell me if there's a couple you're interested in placing your baby with."

After Julia is asleep, we look through the album together. Self-portraits of seven childless couples. His arm is always around her shoulder, in their suburban ranch home, their apartment, their condo, their golden retriever running on the lawn, or their cat on the windowsill. Accompanying each picture is a personal statement, typed or handwritten to an unknown birth mother, promising a loving home, a religious foundation, a solid education.

Eleven years earlier, Brad and I had a page of this scrapbook. We didn't have a dog or cat or lawn, but we had the photo with Brad's arm draped around my shoulder, and the personal statement trying to win over an anonymous pregnant woman. We tried to spin our freelance orchestra conductor and performance artist careers in the most positive light, so we'd be competitive with the equally childless but more financially stable stockbrokers in the album. Lucky for us, Zoe wanted her baby to be raised by artists, and chose us from a Spence-Chapin album just like the one Michael and I are flipping through right now.

Michael and I are casting agents, auditioning these couples for the roles of Best Mommy and Daddy. We read their sentimental statements, look at their affectionate smiles. They look like nice people. But this job of shopping for parents by catalog seems insane.

Michael asks, "Which couple do you think would be the best parents?"

There are teachers, investment bankers, gardeners, and homemakers. They are homely, attractive, fat, thin. They are good writers and terrible writers. They all desperately want a baby. I turn the pages of the album again, pausing at each portrait to imagine the couple holding this baby inside me.

"We are," I say.

"Yes!" Michael groans in relief.

"These people don't know how to raise a lesbian athlete," I say. "We do."

"Exactly!"

This is suddenly all too ridiculous. I feel bad for the childless couples. I hope Spence-Chapin shows their snapshots to the right pregnant casting agents and they all land dream roles as mommies and daddies. Michael and I laugh till we're falling over each other on the sofa, like we're drunk. We're laughing and kissing, and I'm crying at the same time. My peals of laughter sound an awful lot like screaming, because, damn it, that's just the way I am these days. Julia wakes up and staggers into the living room with bleary eyes, wanting to know what's making us laugh like maniacs.

This is the first moment since showing Michael the sonogram image of the baby that I feel like we're together in this journey again. We've got each other. Michael and I can raise this child together. Julia will have a little sister. Michael and I will get married and we'll be a family. Maybe I'm even a little bit happy. That scares me.

Tuh! Tuh! Tuh!

"We're the best parents, *unless* the baby is sick or handicapped," I say to Michael, after Julia is back in bed. "That's the deal breaker. Then we'll give the baby up for adoption, to special needs adoption."

Now we're both good and unhappy again, and safely out of range of the Evil Eye.

Michael hears me but doesn't say anything. He nods. I interpret his nod as an agreement that we will give up the baby for adoption if it's handicapped or sick. I've probably misinterpreted his nod. It's more likely that he's angry with me, but he's in no mood to talk about it.

What I Know

1. I'm going to have this baby.
2. We're going to keep it. . . .
3. Unless there's something wrong with it. . . . I think.

I call Spence-Chapin to tell them my decision. Sasha the social worker knows about birth mothers. She tells me I might change my mind, even if the baby is healthy. The agency can place the newborn baby with foster parents while I decide. But that's crazy, I think. How can I decide, if the baby is with someone else? How can I nurse the baby if the baby is with foster parents? We're going to keep the baby. She accepts my decision as conditional, assures us that my file is active and that I can change my mind at any time before or after the baby is born.

"Do you want to have a contingency plan in place in case the baby is handicapped?" she asks. I don't know. Maybe. They are prepared to place the baby in a foster home, find an adoptive family, if I change my mind. They will, if I need, pay for my prenatal care, my food and rent. They will pay for baby clothes and doctors bills if I need.

Wow! I am overwhelmed by the abundance of their offerings, and realize that Zoe benefited from their professional generosity nine years ago. I don't feel I deserve it. I'm a grown-up, not a pregnant teenager; I have a home and health insurance—albeit crappy health insurance—a family who cares for me. I have Michael. I thank her, but decline. I decide to contribute money to Spence-Chapin when I have a regular income again.

Lamaze: Second Lesson

"So a lady says to me, 'After my baby is born, is there anything I should seek to avoid?' And I say, 'Yes—pregnancy.' So . . . Michael and Alice, you're going to have a baby!" Joy teaches us Lamaze breathing technique. She explains what an Apgar score is—the report card for the newborn, a number from zero (very bad) to ten (very good) that indicates the infant's general health at birth.

"Here's a tip for you, Michael. Fathers always try to be helpful in the delivery room, but don't take it personally when she treats you horrible during labor. You won't recognize her. She'll insult you. I'm not kidding, she'll act like you're not there, she'll call you horrible things, she'll talk like a sailor. Remember, she's not Alice anymore, she's a woman in labor. Hang in there. Now I want you to watch this videotape together before my next visit. So long, you guys."

Since I'm grounded for three months, Joy's entertaining visits to our living room are like date nights for me and Michael. Tonight we get a double feature—Joy's comedy act followed by a movie. We watch it while Julia sleeps. It's pure propaganda. Three women give birth, with supportive husbands nearby, and without much pain. One woman is low-key with long wavy blond hair, one woman is perky and has a black Afro, one is shy and has curly red hair. At least there are some contrasts in hairstyle. The low-key blond gives birth as if she's in a yoga class. Her meditative state is amped up with heavy breathing when she's pushing, like she's demonstrating Kundalini Breath of Fire. When the black lady gives birth, it sounds like she's having a fabulous orgasm. The red-haired lady calmly narrates her fears throughout the process, and tells the camera in an even-tone voice, "This hurts a great deal." Lamaze technique wins the day—Hurrah!

Solo Theater

My students are beginning to perform their solos for the class.

Jeremiah: "I remember Alabama summers. Yearning to patty cake with the sun. Uncle raped my sister at twelve in the front seat of the '76 Mustang."

Bella: "He holds the guitar quiet like water."

Kayla: "I remember walking through the projects in my Corpus Christi uniform, my Uncle Tom Uniform. I'm twelve years old. My friend can't sleep over because I live in the projects."

Dani Athena, the forty-something choreographer and high school dance teacher, works without text. She arranges clumps of moss and dirt as her stage set, turns off the overhead lights, and lights a candle. In the dark she performs a mysterious dance and monologue that we collectively understand is about dying.

After class, Dani asks if I can meet for a few minutes. "I

want to talk to you about my piece, but I don't want to share this with the class. It will be useful for you to know, as my teacher, that . . . I have rectal cancer, and I just found out this week that it's metastasized to my liver. I've decided not to do chemo or radiation, because it will just prolong my life a few months, but it would really diminish my quality of life. My doctor thinks I have less than a year left. I don't want the class to know, but I want you to know so you can help me finish this piece."

"How can I support you in class? What would be most valuable to you?"

"Just coming here, being with this group, showing new material every week, knowing that you know what the piece is about and that you'll help me shape it. That's enough."

She hugs me. Her flexible dancer's body accommodates to my pregnant roundness. I wrap my arms around her thin back. Her angular face rests on my soft cheek. We breathe together, and I think I feel three hearts beating—mine and Dani's, beating side-by-side in unison, and the faster heartbeat of my mysterious daughter, waiting with surprising patience to be born, Dani Athena so filled with life I think hers can't be extinguished.

"What's the most frightening thing for you?"

"I'm scared of physical pain. I'm scared of running out of time. I'm not afraid of dying."

Dani Athena is the most generous person in the room. She is awed by the work of the other students, and they light up when she gives them feedback. Her own performances frighten, hypnotize, and ignite the class. Her mysterious choreography and props, imported from the natural world, transforms the ordinariness of the sterile classroom. Following her lead, the other students risk making solo works that they don't immediately understand.

I am humbled by Dani, by our parallel secrets. I'm expecting a baby, and I'm terrified. She is dying, but she's not scared. She embraces this journey toward death as an adventure. She keeps looking for opportunities to give and give and give, before she runs out of time. I want to be more like Dani. I pay careful attention to her, to her optimism and her generosity, the way the class lights up when she talks to them, when she performs. Emulating her makes me a better teacher. I carefully prepare my classes with the needs of each student in mind. The class is doing remarkable work. I help Dani shape her piece.

I cab home from The New School each Monday and crawl back into bed. I close my eyes and try to preserve in me, for as long as I can, the connection I feel to my students. I savor Dani Athena's life-affirming generosity. I sleep. When I awake there's the old pessimism.

Lamaze: Third Lesson

"I saved the best for last," says Joy on her final Tuesday night visit. "Drumroll, please—The disaster scenarios! I always say to expectant moms, this lesson could save your life, okay? So listen up."

Joy has spent the first thirty minutes of the lesson leading us through a practice session of Lamaze breathing and relaxation technique. We stop relaxing as Joy sets up her flip chart and turns to the page showing all the things that can go wrong—disastrously, fatally wrong, at the last moment.

"You are a prime candidate," she cheerfully assures me, "for the most dangerous of these complications—hemorrhaging. Why do you think all those pioneer women died in childbirth? They bled to death! You think that doesn't happen anymore? Wrong! They'd like you to think it doesn't happen, not in this day and age, right? Dying in childbirth only happens in third world countries, right? Not! Happens all the time. Right here, New York City, even in New York Hospital Cornell Medical Center. I'm a nurse in the neonatal unit. You wouldn't believe what I see. Just last week—I probably shouldn't tell you this—but anyway, just last week, a pregnant lady starts to bleed, so she calls an ambulance, and she's heading over in the ambulance but they can't stop the bleeding and by the time they get to the hospital—I really shouldn't tell you this—she's dead on arrival. And they can't save the baby.

"Human women are very poorly designed for childbirth. There's not enough room. Okay, look at this chart: female anatomy. Stupid design. What was God thinking when he gave women such a narrow pelvis? Did you ever see a horse give birth? The mare breezes through it, vroom, kaboom, ten minutes and the colt is out of there. Because a horse's pelvis is wider, proportionally, than ours. Jeez, a horse! Just think about that. Think about a colt with its long knobby legs, and she just pushes it out. But no-oo, God wanted humans to stand on two legs, right? so he streamlined us for walking, and consequently our hips are too narrow, and Alice you've got really narrow hips, relative to, well, relative to the size of a baby.

"And let's talk about age. Whew!! I'm sure you've heard the term *advanced maternal age*. You'll be forty-five, right? You don't get much more advanced than that, and if you do, you're on the front page of the tabloids. If this were a hundred years ago and you were pregnant at forty-five . . . well, a hundred years ago, if you were forty-five, you'd be dead! Nature didn't intend the human body to be pregnant or even alive at forty-five, you see, so this is not a normal thing. And of course advanced maternal age increases the risk of hemorrhaging. A lot!

"Plus, you're a DES daughter, and that increases the risk of hemorrhaging even more. And you've got a double uterus, right? That's terrible.

"And the position of your baby, I'm afraid, *placenta previa*—Whoa, Nellie, couldn't be worse. That's the worst. The! Worst! The baby could just pull away from the placenta and—BOOM!—there you are, bleeding uncontrollably, like that lady in the ambulance I told you about. You've got every possible risk factor. You're like the perfect storm! So listen up, if you start bleeding, call an ambulance! Don't wait to see if the bleeding stops, just call instantly. Promise me that.

"C'mon, don't look so worried. You'll be fine. You know me, I'm a performer like you, remember? At least I got your attention, right? Cheer her up, Michael, I gotta go. Nice meeting you guys."

Scene 8

A Litigious Mood

I'm the only woman in America who's about to die in childbirth. I know this fear is inflated but it takes hold. It's a genuine phobia.

"You're not going to die in childbirth," says Michael. "Joy likes to get a reaction from her audience and she succeeded. You're going to be fine. The baby will be fine."

"I know," I say, but I don't believe it.

My fear of bleeding to death shouts louder in my head than my fear that I won't be able to love this baby, so my new phobia gives me some relief from my worst fear.

I'm more despondent than ever. I want to give up the baby for adoption again.

"No, Alice," said Michael. "We're not giving the baby up for adoption."

"I don't think I can be a good parent if the baby is sick or deformed. I can't do it, Michael."

"Of course you can."

"We don't make enough money to raise a baby with special

needs. We barely make ends meet as it is, even when I'm not on bed rest. I don't want to do it."

Michael, his superhuman patience finally at its limit, looks at me with a cross of pity and disdain. He ignores this outburst. He is accustomed to the perpetually changing mind and fluctuating emotions of his pregnant fiancée.

I'm in a litigious mood. We're going to need money to raise this baby, whether it's sick or not, whether I die in childbirth or not. There was clearly medical malpractice. Can I sue Robin? She insisted I was in menopause, even after doing an internal exam when I was five months pregnant. She's a good person, I've always liked her. But she screwed up. I call a lawyer I know from Julia's school. She gives me a list of medical malpractice lawyers she knows. Lying in bed on my left side, between naps, editing, drinking blue Gatorade, I call lawyers.

"These cases never amount to anything," says the first guy I called. "I took one of them before, worked on it for two years, and lost a bundle of money. Good luck to you and your baby, but I never take these cases anymore."

A second lawyer says the same thing.

The third lawyer tells me to call back after the baby is born, when I know what damages, if any, I will be suing for. "Meanwhile," she advises, "keep careful notes."

What I Know

1. I'm going to have a baby in two months, maybe sooner.
2. It will be a girl, probably. . . .
3. With a fatal disorder and a penis, maybe.
4. An athletic lesbian, maybe.
5. She might have surgery to disguise her penis as a clitoris, or maybe we'll leave the penis as a penis.
6. I'll die in childbirth, I think.
7. She may be adopted by a Christian, evangelical, homophobic family, which will tolerate neither her lesbianism nor her penis.
8. This should be more than enough worry to ward off the Evil Eye.
9. *Tuh! Tuh! Tuh!*

Scene 9

December

It's December 1. My birthday was a week ago. I'm forty-five. Julia and Michael baked a cake for me. My due date is December 25, or December 11 or 29 or January 1 or 7. It's hard to get an accurate due date in the twenty-sixth week of pregnancy, but I've certainly passed the important pregnancy landmark of thirty-two weeks. I've been lying on my left side for two and a half months. Remarkably, I haven't given birth prematurely. It would be safe to give birth now, at eight months or so. The lungs are developed, and the heart is strong. I'm going to have a baby soon.

There's been a constant talk on the radio about the dreaded, ticking clock of Y2K. The industrial and digital world will grind to a halt at midnight, on December 31, 1999, as it rolls over to Year 2000, because the world's computer infrastructure is predicated on twentieth-century numeration, and will not compute the change to the twenty-first century. Given my luck, I'll go into labor on December 31, the power will go out at midnight, and I'll need an emergency C-section, by candlelight, in an unheated hospital room in the middle of winter, while I bleed to death.

* * *

My sisters ask me if I want to have a baby shower.

This is a trick question. I don't want to have a baby, so I don't want a baby shower. I don't want anyone to know I'm having a baby, because then it's really happening, so I don't want a baby shower. I might be giving up the baby for adoption, so I don't want a baby shower—cause, heck, what's the etiquette? Who gets to keep the presents? Do I send the rattles and board books and stuffed animals to the adoptive parents?

And do the guests bring pink or blue gifts? The baby might be a girl with a penis, or a boy with two X chromosomes. She might have her penis turned into a clitoris with her mile-long sexual nerve neatly folded up and tucked away in her little jewel bag, or he might grow up to be a radical lesbian hermaphrodite transgender lobbyist athlete. She might have to be raced to the emergency room to get her enzyme treatment so she doesn't turn into a pillar of salt, or a salt-wasted pillow.

I'm having a baby. I'm not having an abortion. I'm not going to give birth prematurely. I'm not going to give this baby up for adoption, unless . . . oh, never mind. I'm having a baby. It's not going to stay inside of me forever. I think I'm going to have the baby very soon. It makes me lonely. For me. For the baby. Hardly anybody knows about it. I've been indoors on my left side since I found out I was pregnant, so hardly anyone has seen me pregnant. Strangers on the street haven't asked me when I'm due. My mother isn't alive, my father lives far away. I haven't been taking prenatal exercise classes with other expectant moms. I have been too depressed and too indecisive and too horrified and too guilty about my feelings to call anybody. I've isolated myself. I've asked my few friends who know I'm pregnant to keep it a secret. I'll have to come out of the closet sooner or later, either as a new mother with a new baby, or as a new mother who has given away her new baby.

Yes, I do want to have a baby shower.

My new friend Susan Feiner, mother of Julia's friend Sophie from Hebrew class, will host the shower at her beautiful Upper West Side apartment. I give my sisters a list of my women friends. Most of them will be surprised to hear that I'm pregnant. Madeline wants to postpone the party till later in December, because of her busy work schedule, but my body is telling me I'm going to have this baby really, really soon, so I persuade my sisters to schedule it for next week, the second Saturday in December.

Solo Theater

My students liberate one another from the literal. Dani's radical performance imagery has raised the stakes for the class. She has inspired them. I have inspired them. They are moved by our parallel secrets—the invisible, imminent life and the invisible, imminent death in the room.

"Finding the story you want to tell is only the beginning," I tell them. "There are countless ways to tell a story. You have to find the way to tell your story. If you're lucky, your story will guide you."

Bella: "I ran away when I was two. I'm Lizard. Are you my grandma?"

Dani: "Put your head on this moss. You are my song."

Miriam: "Tea has been ready for almost thirty years. Grandma has wrinkles you could swim in."

Telling the Story

Michael's mother tells the story this way. "It's a miracle baby. It's God's miracle. Thank you, Jesus Christ."

Julia tells it this way. "My parents adopted me because my mom's doctor said she could never get pregnant. But her doctor was wrong, and now I'm going to have a baby sister or brother!"

Michael tells it this way. "I didn't expect to have a child with Alice. I'm so happy we are."

The neighborhood gossip version. "She couldn't get pregnant with her first husband, but Michael has really good aim."

My dad's version. "Now you'll finally know what it's like to be a real mother."

Or Dylan's version. "I can tell from your sexual glow that you're pregnant."

A dozen doctors' divergent versions: This is the story of . . .

your infertility

your early menopause

your underwire bra

your middle-aged loss of muscle tone

your atrophied bladder

your large tumor

your emergency CAT scan

the story of "we found something in you; we found a baby"

the story of the girl with a penis

the girl without a penis

the girl whose penis I can carve and mold into a clitoris

the girl who would grow up to be a lesbian, athletic, transgender activist, enraged that her penis had been mutilated to resemble a clitoris

the story of . . .

the late term abortion

being stoned by right-to-life protesters in Wichita

a five-day labor to deliver a dead, dismembered fetus

the healthy baby who was given up for adoption to the corpulent couple on Long Island with the golden retriever in the front yard

the sick baby who was given up for adoption to an evangelical Christian family in Salt Lake City

the ten-page story I wrote to persuade a medical malpractice lawyer to take my case.

Baby Shower

The morning of the baby shower, I go stark raving mad.

That's what they say in fairy tales, when the evil kings and queens and lonely witches and demons and Rumpelstiltskins become the story's losers.

I wake up in the dark with a panic attack, sweating and hyperventilating. The baby shower is today. I have to face my women friends, and have them see me for the first time. My pregnancy was hidden from me for the first six months. For the last three months, I've hidden my pregnancy from the outside world. They don't know that I neglected the baby, that I subjected it to terrible things, that I've wanted to abort the baby, give it away. All that sturm und drang has taken place in a hermetically sealed world that includes only my immediate family, a slew of doctors, a hyperactive birthing coach, an adoption social worker, and a receptionist at the Wichita Women's Health Center.

My belly is now huge.

I am going to the gallows.

They'll laugh at me for being so foolish.

They'll pity me for being so miserable.

They'll stone me for being so hateful.

Worst of all, there will be no turning back.

Showing up at my baby shower is signing a contract to be this baby's mother.

At six in the morning I go stark raving mad. I wake up hyperventilating and then screaming and shaking. Michael holds me.

Then it stopped as suddenly as it started.

It was time to go to a party.

I got dressed in the black, Indian cotton shirt my writer friend Patty gave me. She would be there.

I put on the necklace my sisters Madeline and Jennifer gave me. They would be there.

I helped Julia get dressed in her blue party dress.

It was a great party.

I was finally coming out as a pregnant woman. I had to cram nine months of pregnancy into one afternoon. What was I thinking for the past three months? Why hadn't I called on my friends? Here they were, happy for me, for my family. It was the most natural thing. I was having a baby, and my friends and family were there to celebrate with me.

It was heaven having my wonderful women friends all together. From grad school, college, friends from Julia's elementary and pre-schools, theater and writing friends, my sisters. It was fun to sit upright all afternoon, and not have to lie down on my left side and drink Gatorade. It was fun to open presents. The three children, Julia and Sophie and Ben, were in charge of organizing the presents, which included lots of giggling and oceans of tissue paper. My friends were happy for me. I was out of the closet, I was accepting gifts for the baby, I was welcoming my friends' congratulations.

It was the most natural thing in the world.

It was the happiest I'd been in nine months.

It was magnificently ordinary.

It was a baby shower.

It was a great party.

I was so happy.

Tuh! Tuh! Tuh! Don't tempt the Evil Eye.

Terror in the pit of my stomach. I'd thrown away the key to the escape hatch.

Solo Theater

There are only two more classes in the semester. Remarkably I haven't missed a single class. Tonight is the rehearsal for the final performance next Monday. It will be an informal performance in a small studio theater at The New School. Each student will perform ten minutes of his or her original solo work-in-progress, for an invited audience of friends.

After the rehearsal is over, I ask my students, "Why do people make theater? Why do you want to perform, and for whom?"

Dani: "My performance is a gift for the class."

Miriam: "I'm going to invite my extended family over for dinner and make them watch my solo show about my two grandmothers arguing over tea in heaven. After I perform, I won't let them out till everybody puts this dumb feud to rest."

Kayla: "I want to perform my piece for inner city black teens and for rich suburban white teens at the same time—Yeah, right. In my dreams."

Jeremiah: "I'll perform this everywhere, for everyone who will listen to me."

At Dr. Rosenbloom's insistence, I switch to a new doctor she recommended, at New York Hospital's obstetrics clinic. "If the baby has medical problems, your insurance won't cover it unless your doctor is in-network. You could incur costs you would never be able to pay off in your entire life."

I like my new, in-network doctor, Barbara. I don't have to tell her the whole story. She treats me like a regular pregnant woman, with no extra drama. She's warm, confident. She speaks about my baby with great affection. I feel safe with her.

"It's getting close to your due date, and you haven't begun to dilate. We should be seeing some action down there. I want you to get out of bed and walk. Have sex if you want. Get things moving. This is it, the final stretch."

I cup my left hand underneath my huge belly to support it, so it will hurt less. Walking a block feels like running a marathon. I get winded after a few steps and have to stop and rest. It's thrilling and scary to be out of the apartment, making small talk with strangers and acquaintances, parents from Julia's school, store owners who haven't seen me all fall. I accept congratulations and pats on my belly.

Later, when Julia is asleep, I tell Michael, "My doctor says we can have sex . . . if you're interested."

"I'm very interested!"

We haven't made love for three months. We're out of practice and my belly keeps getting in the way, creating comic logistical challenges, until we assume the classic spoon position. It's breathtaking and kind of scary when he enters me, and I'm soon transported into pregnancy-hormone-enhanced ecstasy. I lie in Michael's arms in post-coital bliss.

"I kept thinking, 'I'm going to push the baby out with my orgasms.'"

"And I kept thinking, 'What if I'm poking the baby in the eye with my penis?'"

"No, you didn't think that."

"Yes, I did. I was worried my penis was poking her in the eye."

The next moment we're laughing our heads off, and I can't decide which I love more, laughing with Michael or making love with him, and I'm so glad I don't have to choose. I hope our baby will share our goofball sense of humor. Our laughter wakes Julia, and we cover ourselves with a blanket just in time, as she staggers into our room bleary-eyed to find out what's so funny.

Scene 10

Labor

Sunday morning, after two days off bed rest, I woke up at 6:30 a.m. with contractions every five minutes.

This was going to be okay. I didn't know what would happen the day after the birth, but this was today, I knew exactly what was going to happen and what I was going to do. I wasn't waffling or ambivalent, thinking of alternatives and ways of backing out. I was absolutely clear that I was going to have this baby. It was December 11, not December 31. I wouldn't have to face the Y2K global meltdown.

We hadn't chosen a name yet, because we couldn't agree on one. We had agreed to choose a name after the baby was born.

Tomorrow was my solo theater students' end-of-semester performance. I asked my substitute to cover.

I called Barbara. Alas, today and tomorrow were her days off. I was assigned Dr. Tara Carson—a gorgeous young doctor whom Michael and I had met at the clinic's open house. Tara had chatted with us at the open house, and made us both nervous when she bragged that she was dating a New York Mets pitcher, and had stayed out partying all night before working a two-day shift. All the doctors at the New York Hospital obstetrics department looked like glamorous TV actors—understudies for the cast of *ER.* Tara would be appearing tonight in the role of my ob-gyn.

Per Tara's instructions, I called her with updates on the contractions throughout the day. She told me to spend Sunday night at home and come in Monday, or when the contractions were really hurting, whichever came first. Michael brought Julia over to Sophie's, where Susan and Mark would take care of her.

I had a sleepless night—every contraction woke me. Monday at sunrise the contractions were quite painful. Michael and I cabbed to New York Hospital on York Avenue and Sixty-seventh Street.

"Your cervix hasn't even begun to dilate," Tara scolded, as if I hadn't turned in my homework on time. Without warning, she dilated me by hand, using her fingers to stretch open the os, the hole in the cervix.

"OW! OW! THAT HURTS," I screamed, as I felt my cervix ripping.

"You ain't seen nothing yet. Now you guys walk back to the West Side, and keep walking. You got to get this thing moving. You're nowhere near ready to deliver. Don't come back until the contractions hurt so much you can't stand it anymore."

We walked the width of Manhattan, from the hospital by the East River, to Riverside Park on the Hudson River. Every few minutes, as a contraction rolled through, I groaned and doubled over, using Michael's shoulder for support. We walked in Riverside Park, with a halting rhythm—walk, contraction, groan, double over, walk, contraction, groan, double over—punctuated by conversations with curious and congratulatory passersby, my spontaneous nosebleed, and a sunset over New Jersey.

We went to a coffee shop on Broadway for dinner, an absurd place to be in labor but Michael was very hungry, and in the ever-shorter moments between contractions, so was I. Squeezed into our booth at Café 83, with barely room for my stomach, I tried to silence my groans during contractions, between bites of a cheeseburger.

"When are you due?" asked the young blond sitting with her boyfriend at the table next to us.

"RIGHT NOW!" I roared through gritted teeth, gripping the table at an especially intense contraction. The couple quickly paid their check and left.

"You just ended their relationship," Michael teased. "They were probably talking about how much they both want children, but you put the kibosh on that, didn't you?"

Now I was laughing while having a contraction, a bizarre sensation. Michael enjoyed the spectacle, so he kept up a comic monologue while I alternated between laughing and roaring in pain. The biological imperative of going into labor, the adrenalin, the hormones, the cheeseburger, Michael's sense of humor, the absurdity of the situation released me from my obsessive fears.

At six in the evening, when I couldn't stand the pain, we went back to the hospital. I clung to the reception desk, doubled over, as my next contraction reached a new level of intensity.

"That's more like it," said Tara cheerily.

The nurse helped me into a cotton gown and into a high-tech bed, surrounded by machines and monitors. The young Indian anesthesiologist came in to give me an epidural. "I am going to insert a catheter into the space at the bottom of your spine. For one-out-of-a-hundred women, it will feel as though you have been shot in the back with a gun. If that is the case, your left leg will kick involuntarily."

It felt like I was shot in the back with a gun, and my left leg kicked involuntarily. I'm the queen of the one-in-a-hundred chance. I guess dying in childbirth is next. The pain quickly subsided, but the violence of the sensation made my body pessimistic. I distracted myself from this newest trauma by wondering if the baby would have a penis or something penislike. What would it look like? Would it be an entirely new genital shape? Would it be nameable? Would the baby be nameable?

Michael stayed close to me. He charmed the nurses. He held water to my lips when I was thirsty. He stroked my shoulders and held my hand. He talked to me, and stopped talking when I wanted him to stop talking. He was fantastic. I felt entirely distant from him.

"I want to ask you a favor," I said to the nurse. "When the baby is born, please don't say 'It's a boy!' or 'It's a girl.' Dr. Christopoulos, from endocrinology, is going to look at the baby's genitals when it's born. I'd like her to tell me the baby's gender."

The nurse noted this on my chart, in case the next day's nurse switched with her at midnight before the baby was born. I told her I hoped she didn't have to show it to the nurse on the next shift. My contractions had started thirty-six hours ago. I was running out of steam, and I wanted to get it over with.

Things weren't moving as quickly as my doctor wanted. She gave me a drug to induce labor. The epidural started wearing off.

They dripped more into me. I hadn't slept for two days. I hadn't moved for three months—until today when I walked for miles. I watched my contractions on the monitor. Hours passed. The epidural wore off, and it hurt like hell. They dripped more painkiller and I had no awareness of my lower body. It wore off again, so that all I was conscious of was the pain in my lower body. Numb. Pain. Numb. Pain. Numb. Pain. . . . This cycle repeated, part of a polyrhythmic symphony of lights and beeps and contractions, my heartbeat, the baby's heartbeat, my blood pressure tests, the crescendo and decrescendo of pain. Ten hours had passed since the epidural. At four in the morning I asked for a C-section. Tara said no.

The nurse told me to push. Michael told me to push. I couldn't push. I was numb from the waist down. The idea of pushing had no physical meaning for me. I didn't know how or where to push. Tara told the nurse to stop the painkillers. I felt the pain and the baby and the contractions, but I had no strength, and the pain was frightening. I didn't know what I was pushing. My useless attempts to push bore no resemblance to the Lamaze-approved labor of the three women with different-colored hair in the movie.

"I'm going to give you an episiotomy." I heard the snip through flesh. I was sad for my vagina. Two nurses and a doctor and Michael screamed at me to push. "I don't know what to push, I don't know where to push," I cried.

"Push like you're having an enormous bowel movement!" ordered Tara.

I could work with that. I had forty-five-years experience shitting, and my body remembered how to do it, even paralyzed from the waist down. "C'mon, c'mon, harder, like you're having an enormous shit!" No painkiller. "Keep pushing! Just Push Push Push Push Push Push."

At 5:30 a.m., on December 13, 1999, forty-seven hours after the contractions started, I gave birth.

"Umbilical cord's around her neck. . . . She's okay. She's breathing."

ACT III

An Unexpected Life

Scene 1

In Hospital

There was once a poor woodcutter and his wife who had longed for many years for a child. Finally a tiny little girl was born to them. "She's no ordinary child," her father declared when he saw how small she was. "She must have come from the fairy world." His wife nodded as she stroked the tiny form beside her on the pillow. "Why, she's no bigger than your little finger," she said. And from that day the child was known as Little Finger.

—From Little Finger of the Watermelon Patch, *a Vietnamese tale*

There was no cry, no sound.

"APGAR score, four."

"Alice, it's a girl. Her genitals are fine," the nurse said quietly.

That was good to hear.

Michael mopped the sweat from my forehead and hair.

The nurse called out the second APGAR score. Six.

They cleaned the baby, raised the back of my bed, and put her on my chest. Michael perched on the edge of the hospital bed with me, his large hand cradling our baby. I wished we'd chosen a name for her.

She was tiny. Her legs were folded tightly into her belly, making her look smaller still. Her skin was pale. Her red lips formed a miniature rosebud. Her one wisp of hair, wet and matted to her head, was nearly blond. Blue eyes. She had a large forehead and a small, sweet, funny-looking, lopsided face, as if her features had all slid down from her forehead into a puddle near her chin. She was a girl, with tiny, perfectly formed labia. She weighed exactly five pounds.

I was prepared for a penis, but somehow I wasn't prepared for blond. I expected her to look Mediterranean, like me, with darker skin and hair.

I wanted to be in love with this baby. I had hoped for instant love, which would redeem the previous months of not wanting to have a baby. My baby. I was in love with her beautiful rosebud mouth, her impossibly small fingers, which I caressed with my gargantuan fingers. All I wanted was to take care of her, to help her to get strong. I was not instantly in love. Nor was I not in love. She needed a name.

"Why is she so small?" I asked.

"She's not so small," said Tara. "Five pounds is in the normal range."

"Why is her head lopsided?" I said.

"Their heads get squished during childbirth," she said. "All babies look like old men with wrinkled faces when they're just born."

Julia didn't. Brad and I were at Julia's birth. When she was born, she looked perfect. Julia's birth mother, twenty-year-old Zoe, used no painkillers, and she pushed for only thirty minutes. As Julia's head crowned, the Jamaican midwife announced exuberantly, "I see a lot of black hair, I see a lot of black hair." And then glistening, big, strong, beautifully formed Julia flew out of Zoe with her arms over her head, her enormous hands, fingers outstretched, into her new world. Newborn Julia large and robust and aware. Broad cheekbones and dark, wide-awake eyes. Loud crying in her first minute, then lying on Zoe's chest and scrambling for her breast, which she energetically sucked. "Alice and Brad are crying," said Zoe, which we hadn't realized until she said it. I loved Julia instantly without expecting to. Once she was wrapped in swaddling, the nurse handed her to me. Her eyes looked at my face, Brad's face, mine, his, mine, his, preternaturally alert and curious and perceptive. Our friends didn't believe she actually looked at us at such a young age—"Newborn babies' eyes can't focus," they said—but she did.

My new baby was tiny and silent and limp and lopsided.

I wanted to be totally in love with her. I hoped nursing her would bring the love on.

She showed some interest in my breast. When I lay her on my chest, she rooted, moving her mouth in the direction of my nipple. But her mouth was so small and weak, my breast so big and hard, and my nipple so flat that she couldn't get it in her mouth, and she quickly lost interest.

A male attendant wheeled Baby and me into my recovery room—a double, partitioned by a pale green curtain, furnished with a vinyl chair, a plastic bassinet, and a hospital bed. The sterile space was redeemed by a wall of windows. The dawn sun streamed in over the East River, lighting Brooklyn's industrial shoreline, and sky, sky, sky, the clouds still painted pink with the fading sunrise. In the water far below, miniature red tugboats heroically pushed barges twenty times their size. To the south, the Roosevelt Island tram flew back and forth, drawing an arc as it carried early morning commuters from small island to big island.

The attendant transferred me from the gurney to the bed, and we started our new family life.

Everything hurt. My vagina was torn. My body felt as if it had been turned inside out. I had enormous hemorrhoids, like two bunches of large grapes, one bunch ringing the inside of my anus and a second bunch outside. Even on the doughnut-shaped pillow supplied by the hospital, I could barely tolerate sitting for ten minutes while baby-girl Cohen and I made futile attempts at nursing. Every two hours, the nurse gave me painkillers, which dulled the pain and made me groggy and disoriented.

Barbara, back on call, sat on the bed and squeezed my hand. "Your body is traumatized from two days of childbirth. It's very hard to give birth at your age. By nature's calendar, you're a very old woman. Twenty-five-year-olds bounce back very quickly. After thirty-five, every year is exponentially more difficult for the mother's body. It might take you six months to recover."

Dr. Melina Christopoulos from endocrinology sashayed into our room, her white lab coat over a miniskirt, grazing the top of her thigh-high black leather boots. Michael perked up.

"Let's see if she has a penis," she said cheerfully, unwrapping the flannel blanket. "No penis. You have beautiful genitals, baby girl. Look at your perfectly shaped labia. You have a lovely clitoris and a gorgeous vagina!"

Now that's some baby talk. Dr. Christopoulos spent a long time looking at the baby from head to toe.

"Okay, guys, good news. No penis. Was only temporarily androgenization from hormone pills. I'll be in touch with you. Bye-bye." She kissed me and Michael on both cheeks.

The fat, humorless lactation nurse known on the floor as Nipple Nazi marched in and commanded me to nurse.

"We're trying, but it doesn't work."

"Of course it works!" she barked.

"I don't think the baby's getting any milk."

She frowned, muttered something unintelligible, stormed out of the room and returned a minute later with the heavy artillery, in the shape of a refrigerator-sized electric pumping machine. Thirty minutes of pumping yielded a tablespoon of milk and very sore nipples.

"It still isn't working," I said on Nipple Nazi's next visit.

She lunged at me with both fat hands. I thought she was going to choke me. Instead she grabbed my breast, hooked me up again to the electric pump, and turned it up to high. When she saw for herself how incompetent I was, mammarily speaking, she sent for reinforcements.

A young smiley nurse came in and took Baby's vital signs. "Her blood sugar is low. I'll need your permission to bring her to the nursery to bottle-feed her." I signed the permission slip and with some gratitude handed my baby to her. Michael napped in the vinyl chair and I drifted in and out of a drug-induced stupor.

When I woke up I had a roommate, who I watched through the gap in the plastic curtain. A young black woman with a robust newborn who looked like a little boy already, with glistening skin, plump arms, big hands, and a passion for kicking his solid legs in the air while making loud and excited baby noises.

His delighted mother laughed and sang to him, and covered him with kisses.

Smiley Nurse brought back our baby, whose blood sugar was much better after a bottle of formula. She slumped limply in my lap, her fingers, tinier than I'd remembered, tinier than my imagination would allow, wrapped halfway around my big finger with the barest hint of a grip.

Passersby peeked in and made boo-hoo sad-faces. "Preemie?" they asked, and hurried on without waiting for an answer. We had frequent visits from Smiley Nurse, Nipple Nazi, and Birth Certificate Lady, who kept coming by and pressuring us for the completed birth certificate. Miranda was our default name, the only one that Michael, Julia, and I all liked. It was fine last week, but Michael and I agreed that Miranda was not the right name for this baby. "Can we fill in a temporary name for now and change it later?"

"Yes."

Michael reached for the form. The nurse pulled it away. "This has to be filled out by the mother. You're not married, so the name is the mother's legal decision." She handed me the form and waited for me to fill it out.

"Okay, Alice, what's her name?" asked Michael testily, angry at the inequality of our legal relationship to our baby.

"As a placeholder, let's write Miranda. When Julia meets her, we'll choose a name together."

I swallowed two more painkillers and lay down, impatient for the drug to work. The room beginning to swim, I watched Michael hold the baby. She was swaddled tightly in a hospital-issue cotton blanket, white with pale red and blue stripes at the edges. Michael unwrapped the blanket to change her diaper. He wiped her and threw away the soiled, preemie-sized diaper, then lifted her by her ankles and laid a fresh diaper under her bottom. He looked at her naked. Even without the swaddling, she was still folded tightly in the fetal position. Michael touched her toes, gently pressed her knees to straighten her legs. He repeated this a few times.

The narcotic was working. . . . I was drifting into sleep.

"Alice. . . . One of her legs is smaller than the other."

"What?"

"One leg is smaller."

I climbed out of bed. Michael gently pressed her knees down. Her right leg, outstretched, didn't quite reach the ankle of her left leg. It was skinnier than the left leg, proportionally smaller, like it belonged to a different baby, a much smaller baby. I panicked and burst into tears. A nurse came in to see what was wrong. My sister Jennifer arrived at just that moment, to meet her baby niece.

In my drug-induced haze, the ensuing parade of doctors launched an avalanche of medical terms and release forms. Michael had to leave to pick up Julia from school. Jennifer stayed with me.

"Hemihypertrophy . . ." "Hemiatrophy . . ." I heard these two words over and over. Asymmetry. One side abnormally large and one side abnormally small. They didn't know for sure which side was the abnormal length, although it was clear to me that the right leg was the dwarfed one. A slew of specialists examined her and pointed out that it wasn't just her legs; her entire body was asymmetrical. The right hand was tinier than the left, the right arm shorter, the right buttock smaller, her right cheekbone and jawbone smaller than the left. When they asked if I understood what they were saying, I told them I had just taken painkillers and wouldn't remember anything they said. So they talked to Jennifer.

With Jennifer's guidance, I signed release forms. An X-ray of her legs. A CAT scan of her head. An MRI of her whole body. Tests you don't imagine your newborn will have on her first day in the world.

A dour neurologist shook his head and said she'd had a stroke.

An upbeat orthopedic surgeon said she'd be a good candidate for leg length surgery when she was older. He gave us his business card.

The supercilious head pediatrician said she thought the neurologist was completely off base, and there was no way a stroke could have caused this.

After a stroke was ruled out by the MRI, the dour neurologist attributed the asymmetry to my bicornuate uterus, suggesting that the left side of the fetus developed in one compartment of my uterus and the right side of the fetus developed in the other compartment of my uterus.

A geneticist rolled his eyes at everybody and said this was obviously a genetic defect, advanced maternal age the most likely culprit.

"Time to pump!" bellowed Nipple Nazi, rolling in the electric breast pump and parting the sea of doctors.

By the end of the day, when the MRI and CAT scan had come back negative, when the X-ray confirmed the obvious—that one side of her body was a lot shorter than the other—the uneasy consensus was that Baby's abnormality was idiopathic. Jennifer explained to me several times that this meant "without known cause."

As my painkillers wore off, a young, cheerleaderish pediatrician had me sign some forms and promised, "Your daughter is entitled to Early Intervention therapies, a free service provided by the State of New York to babies and toddlers with special needs. Because the hospital identified her special needs at birth, you won't have to go through the application procedure. You're very lucky. It can be an extremely time-consuming process otherwise. And you're lucky you're in New York." She pointed out the window, across the Hudson. "In New Jersey they make you jump through hoops to get services.

"Meanwhile, our team would like to work in tandem with your baby's pediatrician. With your permission, we'd like her to be seen by Dr. Elizabeth Creighton. She's in your neighborhood, she's affiliated with New York Hospital, and she accepts your insurance. We'll make the appointment for you. Your baby's going to be seeing the doctor a lot."

Nipple Nazi thrust Baby to my breast, then denounced us for our mutual incompetence and hooked me to the electric pump, ramming the lever to the highest setting like a deranged scientist in a horror flick.

I kept taking pain meds.

In the late afternoon Jennifer left.

My exuberant roommate and her son were discharged.

Michael was home for the night with Julia. She had spent the previous two nights with her friend Sophie.

Smiley Nurse took my very quiet baby to the nursery to bottle-feed her and monitor her vital signs through the night.

I would spend the night at the hospital alone.

I lay in my bed and cried. The night nurse asked what was wrong. Through gulping sobs I told her.

"I really, really, really wish I could do something. But there's nothing I can do."

I believed her. Everybody who worked in this neonatal ward really, really, really wanted to do everything they could do to keep the babies and the mothers safe and healthy. Usually they were successful, and the babies were born healthy, the mothers recovered, and happy parents took their babies home. But once in a while the babies were not put together properly. Their hearts were outside of their chests, their two eyes were on one side of their face, like a flounder or a Picasso painting, their brain didn't function, their lungs didn't work, or their limbs were different sizes. When the babies were not put together right, the parents were sad and scared, and cried gulping, desperate tears in the middle of the night. But all the king's horses and all the king's men and all the doctors in the hospital couldn't put baby together again. The entire hospital staff of doctors and nurses and janitors and receptionists really, really wished they could do something, but sometimes there was nothing they could do.

Michael brought Julia to the hospital the next morning. Her round cheeks were flushed red with December chill and excitement about meeting her little sister.

Michael put tiny baby into Julia's big, warm hands. "Hello, new baby sister!" she whispered, nuzzling Baby's tiny nose with hers. Then she whirled her around too fast, tripping at the end of her turn, beginning to topple over.

"Careful!" Michael and I shouted, lurching to catch Baby. Julia was having a growth spurt, and with her big feet, she was like an oversized puppy, with a tendency to trip over furniture and drop breakable objects.

"I love you, little baby, little sister, I love you so much!" She kissed Baby's forehead. "Mom, she's so beautiful and she's so little and cute. You're so cute and little."

Julia was oblivious to her sister's deformity, and oblivious to my despair, which was a huge relief to me. Her happiness filled the room. Her euphoria was infectious.

"You're the cutest little baby in the whole wide world."

She plunked down on the vinyl-cushioned window seat, held Baby in her lap, and had a heart-to-heart. "I'm your big sister, Julia, and I'm nine and I'm in fourth grade. Did Mommy tell you that I was so surprised when I found out she was going to have a baby? This is what I was like. I was like, 'Excuse me while I drop dead for a minute.' Like this. Bleh!"

Julia flopped over with Baby. I gasped, while Michael jumped up to catch Baby, just in case Julia dropped her, which she didn't.

"I'm going to have so much fun with you, cutie-head. I'll teach you how to read and how to play soccer. What's her name? Did you guys decide without me?"

*   *   *

We unanimously agreed that this baby was definitely not a Miranda.

"I think her name is Eliana," I said.

"You don't think it's a little bit flowery, a little too pretty?" Michael asked.

"I think it works for her," I said.

Julia said, "Eliana is a good name for her, cause she's the prettiest baby and Eliana is the prettiest name. And we could call her Ellie, which is a really cute nickname for such a little cutie."

"Whatever you want," said Michael.

I thought, but didn't say, that a name meaning "My God Has Answered Me" might serve as a talisman, a magical good luck charm, a perpetual prayer, an expression of gratitude, a way of keeping a higher power close to her. My tiny baby with idiopathic deformities could use a higher power close by. I could use one too, even though I was a committed agnostic. We were a family of agnostics. Even Julia, who was immersed in her Hebrew school studies and Bat Mitzvah preparation, and Michael, the only one in our family who believed that examining one's relationship with God was a priority in life. I was far from certain that there was a higher power, but in that moment I was absolutely certain that my baby and I needed one.

Michael shrugged his shoulders. The name Eliana seemed a bit ornate to him, but this was his new role, adjusting his life and his wishes to please the women in his family.

*   *   *

The hospital changed Miranda to Eliana on all their records, but the birth certificate form had already been mailed to the Department of Records. Her legal name was Miranda. We would have to apply for a legal name change.

"The Birth Certificate Lady said that we could fill in a temporary name and change it later."

"We're so sorry that you were misinformed."

I stayed in the hospital for three nights while they tested Eliana, and while I was monitored—for pain, for vital signs, for depression.

When it was time to leave, Michael dressed Eliana in the zero-to three-month Baby Gap outfit we got at the baby shower. It was pathetically large on her, or she was pathetically small in it. Her arms and legs, lost somewhere in the torso section, didn't begin to reach the sleeves. We bundled her the best we could for the chilly December day, strapped her into the car seat, and checked out of the maternity ward. As the elevator doors opened, we saw the dour neurologist.

"Good luck," he said, lowering his head to avoid our eyes.

"Doctor," I said, "do you think she'll ever be able to walk?"

"We just don't know. That's all I can say," he said, shaking his head as he walked out of the elevator.

"Why did you ask him that?" Michael asked, angrily.

"Because I have to know."

"You don't know any more than you did before you asked him, do you? And now you'll just be more worried. What did you hear him say?"

I shrugged my shoulders. "He said, 'We don't know.'"

"That's right. And that's all he said," said Michael, picking up the car seat with Eliana in it.

I nodded. That's all he said, but what I heard was, "Your daughter may never walk," which I translated into, "Your daughter will probably never walk," which I translated into, "Your daughter might be disabled," which I translated into, "We agreed that if our baby is disabled we will give her up for adoption," which translated into, "I don't know if our baby is disabled, so I don't know if we're going to keep her," which translated into, "Michael will want to keep her, and I will want to give her up for adoption," which translated into, "What is wrong with me? Why can't I love my new baby? I'm despicable." Which translated into a horrifying vision of throwing myself in front of a moving truck.

We waited for a taxi in the chilly afternoon under a thick, white sky. Ahead of us in line were an old man in a wheel chair, a teenage boy on crutches, a young man and woman cuddling their new twins, a middle-aged woman propping up a teetering, ancient man, and a mother holding hands with her bald little girl.

I thought about the day Brad and I brought Julia home from Beth Israel Hospital, in the East Village, nine years earlier. We were planning to say a quick good-bye to Julia's birth mother and pick up four-day-old Julia. Just before we left our apartment, the attending doctor phoned and told us to meet him in his office with our Spence-Chapin social worker.

"I have reason to believe that this baby has Down syndrome," he said when we arrived. "She has slanted eyes and broad cheeks, a simian crease in her palm, and trouble sucking, all indicators of Down syndrome. I know you are the potential adoptive parents, but I cannot let you take this baby home until we have completed genetic testing and you have been counseled on the ramifications of raising a child with Down syndrome."

We signed papers as Julia's foster parents, brought her home that day, waiting for the results of her genetic testing. Brad and I spent three days flip-flopping between wanting to keep her no matter what, and wanting to give her up for adoption if she had Down syndrome. Each morning he and I arrived at opposite conclusions, never in sync with each other. The not-knowing whether we were her parents created a chilling distance between us.

Three days later, the hospital's chief geneticist told us, "I don't know whether this baby will be smart or stupid, but I can tell you conclusively that she does not have Down syndrome."

"But what about the simian crease?" Brad asked.

"She does have a simian crease," he said thoughtfully, tracing the straight line across Julia's palm with his finger. "I have a friend with a simian crease. He teaches at MIT."

"How can we go back to that ecstatic feeling of unconditional love, before it was marred by uncertainty?" I asked Patricia, our adoption social worker.

"You can't. Parenting is not about going back," she said. "Parenting is all about moving forward, and constant, unpredictable change."

Michael, Eliana, and I finally got a taxi, which aggressively thrust its way through the crowded Upper East Side streets, narrowly avoiding wide-load pedestrians padded with shopping bags. The winter city, gaudily dressed for the holidays, winked and twinkled her colorful lights, sang songs and jangled her bells, undulating to the rhythm of her crowded sidewalks. She seduced shoppers into stores with dancing windows, reminding me that Hanukkah and Christmas were next week and that I had to buy presents for Julia. Then the taxi withdrew from the holiday maelstrom and entered Central Park and the gray quiet of its leafless trees.

What I Know

1. My baby is tiny.
2. One leg is shorter than the other.
3. She's quiet.
4. She is having trouble nursing.
5. Nobody knows what's wrong with her.
6. Her name is Eliana.
7. Julia is in love with her.
8. Michael adores her.
9. I would give my life for her.
10. I'm afraid of breaking her.
11. I don't know if she will ever walk.
12. She might be disabled. Therefore:
13. We might be giving her up for adoption. Michael doesn't know I'm thinking this.
14. My body hurts terribly.

Scene 2

Home

In the hospital, my obsessive worries were mitigated by the knowledge that a team of specialists was working around the clock to diagnose and cure my baby's problems.

Out of the hospital, there was nobody to help us. There was no diagnosis. There was no cure. There was just our baby. And us.

At night she woke every two hours. She nursed a little bit. Michael gave her a bottle.

We bought her some clothes at Baby Gap. Preemie clothes were too large. We got the extra small preemie size.

The adoption counselor from Spence-Chapin called. "How are you, Alice? How is the baby?"

"She's . . . she has some problems. Idiopathic. She's very small, and one side is shorter than the other."

"Do you want to consider adoption?"

"I don't know. I don't know, I don't know, I don't know."

"How does Michael feel about it?"

"I don't know. I can't talk to him about it yet."

"If you want, we can place Eliana with a foster family while you make up your mind."

"No, no I can't do that. I have to nurse her. I have to nurse her so that I can give her something, so that I can boost her immune system, no matter what happens. If I'm going to love this baby, I have to start now."

"You said she's not getting much breast milk."

"She's getting a little."

"Okay, Alice, I'll call you again soon to see how you're doing. Feel free to call anytime if there's anything we can do."

In the morning we went to Dr. Creighton, the pediatrician New York Hospital arranged for us.

"We don't take *this* insurance," said the receptionist, holding my offending insurance card at a distance, as if it were a stinking turd.

"I thought you took Oxford."

"Not *this* Oxford. We take Oxford Freedom, but you're on Oxford Liberty. We do *not* take Liberty!"

"The hospital made this appointment for us. Our newborn has health problems."

"I'll see what Dr. Creighton has to say."

Dr. Creighton agreed to see Eliana just that one time at no cost. "She's not effectively nursing, and her blood sugar is low. Here's the phone number of a certified lactation consultant. Call her right away. And of course you'll have to find another doctor. Eliana's going to need a lot of medical attention, and you'll need a better insurance plan."

* * *

"We accept all Oxford plans for current patients, but we are not accepting any new Oxford patients."

"Do you ever make exceptions? I live a block away from your office, my newborn has serious health problems, and we can't find a doctor who will see her."

"Oh, my goodness. Let me check with Dr. Levin. He loves babies. . . . I'm going to put you on hold for a moment. . . . Yes, Dr. Levin would be happy to see your baby. Don't worry about the insurance. I'll call Oxford right now to tell them we're opening the panel for you."

I was good at this job of slashing through red tape for Eliana. Just like I was good at obediently lying on my left side and drinking Gatorade for three months to protect her from premature birth. Maybe my administrative perseverance and my protective instincts could serve as a placeholder while I learned to love her.

Dan Levin was gentle with Eliana, talking to her about everything he was doing. He talked to me and Michael like friends.

"The hospital record says that Eliana's asymmetry is a result of Alice's bicornuate uterus. Does that strike anyone else in the room as, well, absurd? Let's try to get a reasonable diagnosis. And, Alice, if you don't feel better in a week, please call me. Postpartum depression shouldn't go untreated."

We saw Dr. Levin every three days. Each time, the diagnosis he noted on the insurance form was "failure to thrive." Failure to thrive, failure to thrive, failure to thrive.

In Levin's waiting room twice a week, I watched toddlers perfecting their new walking skills in the play area, and I marveled at their good fortune to have legs the same length. While observing these symmetrical children, I found myself unconsciously straightening and pulling on Eliana's shorter leg, as if I could lengthen it if only I applied myself to stretching. Symmetry, which I'd previously taken for granted, now seemed miraculous. It was difficult to imagine how Eliana would ever walk, run, play in a playground, ride a bike, without toppling over, without persistent pain. I pondered bicycle mechanics, engineering in my imagination a bike customized for Eliana's different-length legs. I kept gently tugging Eliana's tiny right foot, wishing her leg longer.

Lena, the lactation specialist, came to our apartment for an evaluation session, eighty-five dollars a pop, not covered by bad Oxford. She looked like a hippy—long blond hair and an ankle-length peasant skirt over big sheepskin boots—but her rap was pure Nipple Nazi. "No bottle feeding. Six months of exclusive breastfeeding!"

While Eliana napped, Lena assured me that she would fix my nursing problems in no time. Then Eliana woke up, and she observed our comical lactating attempts. Eliana licked my flat nipple until she got tired of the unrewarded effort. Lena then hooked me up to an electric breast pump, at which I was an utter udder failure, producing less than an ounce of milk. Uncompromising Lena compromised.

On her second visit, Lactation Lena brought props. She set me up on the sofa and arranged my breasts on a lactation pillow, which circled my waist like an inner tube, pastel-colored illustrations of dishes running away with spoons on the cotton cover. She hung a plastic tube around my neck, to which she attached a syringe full of infant formula. The formula flowed through two thin tubes, which she taped, with paper surgical tape, to the top of each nipple.

I looked and felt ridiculous. Lena lay Eliana down on the flat pillow, facing my right nipple and the milk tube. Eliana contentedly sucked formula through the plastic tube. My hands were free. I could read a newspaper, apply makeup, practice clarinet, tear my hair out. Every now and then, perhaps to make me feel better, Eliana found my nipple and took a polite little swig.

"I thought you said no baby formula for six months."

"In extreme circumstances there's a need for supplementation."

"Are we trying to trick Eliana? She's a very smart baby. She knows these taped-on tubes aren't my nipples, and this isn't my breast milk."

"When there's a basic incompatibility, we have to implement a compromise solution."

"What do you mean by basic incompatibility?"

"I thought it was obvious. By incompatibility, I mean your boobs are huge, your nipples are flat, and Eliana's mouth is tiny. You're anatomically and functionally incompatible with each other, so there's no possible way she's going to get enough nutrition by nursing."

"Then what's the point of this charade? Why don't I just bottle-feed her?"

"Because she's getting some breast milk this way, and the lifelong benefits to her immune system are incalculable."

"Okay, if you say so." I bent over to look at Eliana drinking from the tubes. As I leaned forward, the formula from the tube around my neck spilled on Eliana's head. Eliana didn't seem bothered by the white puddle on her head, but I didn't think we both had to look ridiculous.

"I believe I can speak for Eliana when I say this is very embarrassing for both of us. Are you absolutely sure it's important for me to continue to breastfeed her?"

"Absolutely sure," Lena answered.

Sending out a birth announcement briefly crossed my mind.

Eliana (legal name Miranda),
Born (quite by surprise) December 13, 1999
(after 47 hours of hell,
3 months of bed rest,
and 6 months of medical misjudgment and self-delusion)
4lbs, 15 ounces (after several days of failure to thrive)
19 inches (on the left side)
18 inches (on the right side)
to Michael and Alice
(who by the way are planning to get married on June 11,
but have no time to send out invitations.
If you're getting this birth announcement,
you're probably invited to our wedding,
so please hold the date.)

Julia loved Eliana totally and unconditionally. At nine, she was past the age of sibling rivalry. She raced home from school to play with Eliana, dressing her like a doll (she especially liked putting her in the purple velvet cape and matching slippers I'd received at the baby shower), putting Eliana in her big bed, and surrounding her with stuffed animals. She wanted to give her bottles, change her diaper, burp her, bathe her, read to her. She couldn't wait till we moved the bassinet out of our bedroom so she could share a room with her baby sister. At Saturday morning basketball practice, Julia showed Eliana off to her basketball team, and allowed each girl to take a turn holding her.

Michael loved Eliana totally and unconditionally, though he was terrified of breaking her, dropping her from the changing table, rolling on top of her in his sleep after a nighttime feeding. Michael, who had always been a world-class sleeper, able to sleep through the loudest turbulence, now woke up the instant he heard Eliana cry.

Eliana loved all three of us, totally and unconditionally. Even me, though I didn't deserve it. My feelings for her were dominated by my fear of breaking her, my shame that I'd already broken her in ways I didn't yet know.

I studied Eliana—her rosebud mouth and blue green eyes, her peaceful demeanor and remarkable patience, her soft, cooing voice like the most sublime music. I kissed her broad forehead and her tiny nose. Her beauty and fragility—which I studied as if from a distance, although she was in my arms—reminded me of my insufficiency.

Eliana and I spent New Year's Eve home alone. Julia was in LA with Brad. Michael was performing at a First Night celebration in

New Jersey, filling in for a family show I'd originally been scheduled to perform. The producer was happy to substitute Michael's
solo show *Lagushka: The Russian Frog Princess* for my solo show
The Balinese Frog Prince.

I nursed Eliana, with our hybrid tube-tape-nipple arrange-
ment, while watching New Year's Eve coverage, the frenzied
TV celebration intensified this year by Y2K fears and dreams.
Shortly before midnight, Eliana fell asleep. I was too lonely to
ring in the New Millennium alone, so I watched the ball fall at
Times Square with sleeping Eliana on my chest. "Happy New
Year," I whispered to her.

Solo Theater

My dormant work life awakened in January. Editing, teaching, performing. I was grateful that I didn't have to lie on my left side to edit the new issue of *Play by Play*, and we needed the money, but it was too much, too soon.

My spring semester solo theater class started. Last semester my Monday night class was the highlight of my week—the time when I felt myself to be professionally most alive, creative, engaged. Now, having to trudge downtown in the slush on a frigid Monday night was a pain in the neck. I printed a copy of last semester's curriculum and parroted the lecture and workshop I gave at the first class in September. "My goal is to have each of you find the story you want to tell, and the way you want to . . . blah, blah, blah, blah, blah."

My spring semester students were duds. Maybe they were great and I was the dud. My students were twenty-something and all ego, except for Esther Levine, who was eighty-four years old and all ego. The twenty-somethings wanted to create solo works about their sexual coming-of-age. They annoyed and amused me. Half of them were gay guys, and they wrote plays about coming out to their parents, about their first Gay Pride Day. They imitated one another, resulting in a bland sameness to their lewd stories of homoerotic self-discovery. Eighty-four-year-old Esther Levine imitated the young gay guys and produced her own lewd story of erotic self-discovery, circa 1940. None of my students were particularly talented, but they brought a lot of enthusiasm about their sexuality into the classroom, which was convenient, since I couldn't muster enthusiasm about anything.

The second Sunday in January, I was scheduled to perform my solo family show *The Balinese Frog Prince* at the Bank Street College auditorium. Barbara, my ob-gyn, warned me that my body would need more time to recover. But I so desperately wanted to get back to the work that might make me feel like myself again. All fall, I'd looked forward to this January performance. But as the date approached, I found any excuse to avoid rehearsing, and ultimately persuaded myself that I knew the show so well I didn't need to rehearse.

When the performance date arrived I felt only dread. Instead of the intense and somewhat loopy actor and playwright persona I was accustomed to summoning to my children's shows, I was mired in exhaustion and pessimism. In the dressing room, I discovered that my costume was too tight. I hoped that nobody would show up so the show would be canceled. But there was a full house, children and their parents expecting a poignant and funny performance. The producer had paid me in advance.

I performed the twelve characters of *The Balinese Frog Prince* while watching and judging myself from a distance. "I've always wanted a child," said the Old Farmer's Wife after giving birth to a frog. "We will raise you as if you were a regular little boy." Watching my performance from the ceiling, I derided myself for not being able to love my newborn as fully as the Old Farmer's Wife loved her baby frog. Making an audience laugh had always been a euphoric experience, but the audience's laughter seemed to have nothing to do with me. The bright lights were colorless. The lively audience was lifeless.

When it was over I apologized to the producer for my lackluster performance. He looked surprised and claimed he wasn't aware of a problem. I cabbed home and got in bed, pulling the covers over my head.

I didn't want to perform again. Neither did I want to write again—writing a children's novel or play or picture book required a buoyancy and sense of humor I no longer had. I found little joy this winter in teaching my class. I couldn't imagine ever jogging again—my body was so heavy and stiff, it hurt to move. I was a failure this time around at parenting. I was too depressed to call my friends, and felt too guilty to have intimate conversations with Michael and Julia that might reveal my unforgivable ambivalence.

Our old apartment had impressive water pressure and an illegal showerhead from the pre-water-conservation-law days. The hot rainfall was my five-minute daily escape into torrential forgetfulness.

* * *

Late one night, I broached the adoption question. "Since Eliana is quite possibly handicapped, shouldn't we consider . . ."

The subject didn't achieve the status of a conversation. Michael was furious that I was still contemplating adoption. His angry clarity was an unexpected relief, finally releasing me from the broken record that kept skipping back to the same agonized uncertainty.

The adoption door closed, I called Sasha the social worker to thank her for all her help. I told her we'd made up our mind to keep the baby, promised to make a tax-deductible contribution to Spence-Chapin, and asked her not to call again.

I hung up the phone, closed my eyes, inhaled and exhaled slowly, silently talking myself into believing the obvious, impossible, astonishing truth: "We are a family of four. . . . I have two daughters."

My tiny, emaciated baby Eliana had scoliosis, which made her spine curve to the right like the letter C. Her short right leg might prevent her from ever walking. She was having a hard time eating or growing. In my not-knowing, when she was inside me, I neglected her, harmed her. Now she was so quiet. She demanded nothing but needed everything. I wanted to give her everything she needed, but there was so much I didn't think I could do, so much I used to be able to do, that I hoped I would rediscover someday. What could I do for her? . . . I could . . . I would give my life to protect her. I could do that.

*   *   *

I'd expected breastfeeding to be a great bonding experience, but there were all those dopey tubes and the daily comedy of errors of tape coming off nipples and formula spilling on Eliana's head. Instead, I bonded with Eliana when she napped on my belly, her cheek on my chest, where I imagined her listening to my heartbeat, our bodies completing each other like they had been for nine months. For the duration of the nap, I loved her. It was very simple. If only I could extend that love. That simple, peaceful, unfettered love.

Grandma Daisy

In mid-January, Michael's mother arrived from New Orleans, to help take care of the girls and give me time to work while Michael was in Brussels for a week. He'd canceled all his touring in Eliana's first month, but he was committed to this international conference for Arthur Andersen LLP, the gigantic global accounting firm, which in the last year had become his most consistent freelance client.

We'd visited Daisy several times in her modest home in New Orleans East where Michael grew up, most recently in May when Michael, Julia, and I went to the New Orleans Jazz Fest and I nearly fainted in the heat, unaware that I was pregnant. I was very fond of Daisy, and we were generally tolerant of each other's different worldviews. Michael and I had a running joke that she would surreptitiously try to baptize Julia by sprinkling water on her head when we weren't looking.

I loved Daisy's accent, a blend of her rural Mississippi child-hood and five decades in New Orleans. Michael, who had inten-tionally dropped his New Orleans accent in college to avoid being branded with the stereotypes associated with the Deep South, made fun of my attempts to imitate Daisy's voice.

"My mother doesn't sound like Blanche Dubois."

"To me she does."

Daisy took care of Eliana and Julia while I edited *Play by Play*, which needed a lot of attention for me to get the next issue out on time. I was in a lot of physical pain and sad most of the time—grateful that Daisy let me be quiet and sad for as many hours a day as I needed. She blessed every meal and thanked Jesus for everything, above all for our "miracle baby," but she didn't expect me or Julia to pray with her. I knew that she was aware of some of the tumultuous decisions made and unmade during the pregnancy, and I expected her to judge me. But she didn't—or if she did, she kept it to herself. And as far as I could tell, she didn't try to baptize the girls.

Daisy loved to take care of people. She was exceptionally good with babies. I was feeling clueless in this arena, and I watched her carefully. She knew how to rock Eliana to sleep, just how close to hold Eliana's face when she talked to her, how to wipe away baby shit without irritating her skin. She knew how to play with an infant, a skill I'd forgotten. She sang Eliana lul-labies and folk songs I'd never heard. She sat on the floor and entertained Eliana on her lap while playing board games with Julia.

*   *   *

"How's it working out with Mom?" asked Michael, calling from Belgium.

"She's great. We're all fine. Freezing. How's Belgium?"

"It's a beautiful resort, the food is amazing—I'll bring home some Belgian chocolate. It's surreal how much they spend at these conferences. I used to feel guilty about how much I charged, till I saw a planning budget and realized they spend more on balloons than on my weekly fee. But this is a really hard conference."

Michael was essentially a corporate court jester. I teasingly told him he was like the trickster in traditional rituals, who made fun of the king while simultaneously reinforcing the status quo. His job at these training conferences was to teach Arthur Andersen culture and to lampoon it at the same time, with these absurdly funny, faux-corporate characters he invented. Through his comic monologues and audience participation bits, he illuminated Arthur Andersen culture—from the tax code to the dress code and everything in-between—while skewering the very precepts he instructed his audience to follow. The firm used these training conferences to acculturate new hires and seasoned employees into Arthur Andersen's particular worldview. They appreciated Michael's ability to transform dry information into crowd-pleasing entertainment. His corporate audiences always thought he was hilarious. He was accustomed to being a huge hit.

"It's our first European conference, and we're just figuring out this audience. The first two days totally bombed. All the bits that worked so well in Chicago—the Europeans think it's dumb and American. So we've been adjusting, and we're finally getting it.

"And here's an interesting and unexpected development—one of the partners talked to me last night about possibly joining the firm."

"Is that good?"

"I—think so? Maybe. Yeah, I think so. Wouldn't happen for a while. Not for a year probably. But if it works out, I'd be working out of the New York office. So I'd be home more. I could walk to work."

"Wow. That sounds really . . . complicated. Really good! But complicated. Will you still be Michael if you work for Andersen full time, or will you be like *The Invasion of the Body Snatchers*?"

"Who knows? The last two Januarys I was working in El Paso, creating theater with children of Mexican American migrant farmworkers. How did I end up here?"

"Maybe you could still work in El Paso some of the time."

"Yeah, not likely. But this will be good, working in the New York office. I won't be touring so much. You want me to be home more, right?"

I don't know the answer. Yes, of course I want Michael to be home more. I miss him. I need his help with the girls. I asked him to find work that allowed him to be home more, and he's being incredibly responsive and responsible. But will *real* Michael—funny, cynical, ethical, penniless-by-choice, loner, edgy Michael—survive, or will he be selling his soul to the company, replaying the life of his dad who worked at an office job he hated for forty years and then died, a scenario Michael has dreaded? I don't know the answer.

"I'd love it if you were home more. I miss you."

"I miss you and the girls a lot."

*   *   *

Daisy walked Julia to school each morning and forged instant friendships with moms in the school yard and with every shopkeeper in a three-block radius, which was as far as she traveled in New York City. She would have enjoyed being a more adventurous tourist, but she was ill-equipped by wardrobe and by constitution for the cold. By midweek, there were five inches of snow on the ground and the windchill was below zero. Daisy walked through an icy wind to the department store three blocks away and came home with the first wool coat and flannel nightgown she had ever owned.

At the end of the frigid week, Daisy came down with a terrible cold. I gave her hot tea and chicken soup and Advil, and helped her get a cab back to the airport. She had to take care of her ailing sister in Mississippi and her grandbabies in St. Louis.

"I'll see y'all in June!" she said.

Home Remedies

"I have a gift for you," said my friend Sue Schulman. "I've arranged for my yoga teacher to give you private yoga classes at home."

Parvati was her Sanskrit name. She was small, slim, and muscular, about thirty years old, with close-cropped black hair, black lashes, pale skin, and velvety lips—incredibly sexy. It took me by surprise, not that I was attracted to a woman, but that I had any sexual feelings at all. I watched her take off her puffy down jacket and several layers of oversized sweaters, revealing her lithe body in a tank top and sweatpants. There was a lot of touching in my yoga sessions. In my postpregnancy, post-three months of bed rest, post-forty-seven-hours-of-labor, still anemic state, my body was a foreign thing. Before the pregnancy, I'd been strong and flexible. Now my muscles were atrophied and stiff. My body still hurt.

Parvati was gentle but forceful, pressing her body on mine while I was standing, sitting, lying down, using her weight to stretch my legs, my back, my shoulders. I told Parvati, Sue, and Michael that the yoga was restoring my sense of physical well-being. I didn't mention that it was reawakening my libido. I loved her smell, the feel of her hair on my skin when she stood behind me and positioned my pelvis, my shoulders, my neck. The yoga positions were quite painful, but she was intent upon activating my dormant body.

For one hour a week, I practiced yoga poses, which I allowed myself to think of as Parvati embraces. Between her visits, I practiced on my own. Each time I saw her she pressed me into deeper bends, opened my legs in wider stretches.

Eliana was also promised home visits from personal trainers, compliments of New York State's Early Intervention Program.

On a blustery January day, Michael and I took Eliana to be evaluated for services, at the Upper East Side office of Stepping Stone Day School, our Early Intervention administrator. She lay on a gym mat strewn with baby toys, surrounded by a team of five therapists and social workers who carefully observed her and took copious notes. So much attention focused on such a tiny baby! The disparity in cubic space occupied by the observers and the observed was remarkable.

Eliana did what babies do: Reach. Grasp. Look. Make sounds. Then, one by one, the therapists did what Early Intervention evaluators do: Move a toy from side to side, three inches from her face; make eye contact; put a finger in her palm; put a finger in her mouth.

Michael and I held our breath when the cognition specialist spoke. "Eliana presents as an adorable and alert baby girl. . . . No cognitive delays. . . . Educational services are not needed."

Michael and I exhaled.

The other therapists had more complicated diagnoses and goals. They reminded me of the good fairies surrounding newborn Sleeping Beauty's bed, trying to counteract the damage caused by the Evil Fairy, who wished for Baby to prick her finger on a spinning wheel and die. Eliana's evaluators waved their wands and made wishes that would offset the less-than-perfect hand Eliana had been dealt.

"I wish you a straight spine!" said the physical therapy evaluator. (Anyway, that was how I understood her Latin-infused, anatomy-textbook shop-talk about correcting Eliana's scoliosis and minimizing skeletal damage resulting from her asymmetry.)

"I wish you a better suck and a stronger tongue!" (my rough translation), said the speech, language, oral motor, and feeding therapy evaluator, after withdrawing her rubber-gloved finger from Eliana's mouth.

They sent us home with written reports: "Eliana presents as an adorable baby girl with a C-curve from her longer (left) to her shorter (right) side, and severe scoliosis," wrote the physical therapist. "Eliana presents as an adorable baby girl with evidence of palsy on the right side of her face, which interferes with oral motor functioning, nursing of most immediate concern," wrote the speech, language, oral motor, and feeding therapist. Three therapists would be assigned to her case. Home visits from the physical therapist and oral motor therapist would begin in a month.

The ubiquitous "Eliana presents as an adorable baby girl" appeared on every doctor's and therapist's report Michael and I read, often followed by "failure to thrive." I thought Eliana was adorable, but I doubted that adorableness was an objectively observable quality. Did "adorable" carry any useful medical information? I suspected it was the scrap thrown to anxious parents, hungry for good news, any good news, about their special needs child. "Adorable" was comfort food for a starving parental ego.

A Diagnosis

When Eliana was four weeks old, Dr. Melina Christopoulos, the miniskirted endocrinologist, called us.

"I'd like you to come in and meet my colleague Dr. Abigail Arbogast. When I examined Eliana on day she was born, I noticed that she had some unusual features I think Dr. Arbogast would be interested in seeing. I will make point of being there. It will be nice to see you."

Dr. Arbogast left us in the waiting room for three hours, so we were feeling somewhat defensive going in, even though Dr. Christopoulos visited us periodically, wearing a red leather miniskirt and matching thigh-high boots.

"This baby has all of the CLASSIC Russell-Silver syndrome features. Lookit that! Doctor Christopoulos, do ya see those curved PINKY FINGERS! Lookit the small EARS, wouldja lookit that pointy CHIN. . . ."

Dr. Arbogast wore cowboy boots, a denim skirt, and a string

tie with a turquoise pendant over her denim shirt. Her Texas accent completed the middle-aged cowgirl effect.

"And look at this leg length DISCREPANCY. That is the most EXTREME ASYMMETRY I have ever, ever seen on a Russell-Silver child. Usually you don't notice the asymmetry till they're older. Wouldja look at this baby lyin' on her back, she is shaped like a *C*, a classic C-curve as a result of her asymmetry. This is quite remarkable. Yes! Unmistakable!

"Mom, Dad, your baby, Elayna, has Russell-Silver SYNDROME."

"So we gathered," said Michael.

"I am very pleased that you brought her to me. I am an expert on Russell-Silver syndrome. I have patients with Russell-Silver syndrome who come to see me from around the world. The little girl who you passed when you were walking in, she and her family fly in to see me from Michigan several times a year. You're gonna bring Elayna to see me every month. Do you realize, Mom and Dad, how lucky you are to have little Elayna—"

"It's Eliana," Michael corrected her.

"Do you know how lucky you are that Elayna has been diagnosed at such a young age? There are some RSS children who are not diagnosed till they're seven or eight months old, and by then a great deal of damage has already been done."

"What kind of damage?" asked Michael.

Dr. Arbogast answered Michael's question with relish. She relished everything about Russell-Silver syndrome, every gosh darn little bit of it.

"These children have digestive difficulties, you see. They are unable to eat, utterly UNABLE, because they have such severe

REFLUX that they develop EATING AVERSIONS. And you see, these Russell-Silver children would rather STARVE to death than take nourishment. For many of my patients, the only way to nourish them is through a FEEDING TUBE, so we operate on them as babies or as toddlers, and if they won't eat by day, we put that food into their BELLIES at night through a FEEDING TUBE. Which is why I am so PLEASED that Dr. Melina Christopoulos here identified ELAYNA at birth, so that we can try to AVOID having to use the feeding TUBE. Dad, what is the matter with your wife?"

"She's having a hard time taking this all in," he said—an understatement, as I was on the verge of falling apart.

"What's so hard to take in, Mom? You've raised a child before. This is no different. You just raise this baby the way you would raise any other baby, just that she's got a DWARFING syndrome, and we'll be giving her growth HORMONES to make her grow, and I think, because her leg length discrepancy is so EXTREME, you'll probably be looking at some leg-lengthening SURGERIES throughout her childhood, which could mean a lot of time in and out of WHEELCHAIRS, but it's worth it, as long as there's no NEUROLOGICAL DAMAGE. And then a lot of these children have LEARNING DISORDERS, nobody knows why but they do, so they tend to go to special schools, and one of my RSS patients is autistic. Dad, what is the matter with your wife?"

"I can't do it," I sobbed.

"Alice, honey, we can figure it out, it's going to be okay."

"No it's not, it's too much. Maybe we should call the adoption agency."

"Let's talk about this at home."

"Don't worry, Alice," purred Dr. Christopoulos. "All she needs is love. It will be fine."

I broke down into loud, stupid tears in Dr. Arbogast's office.

"Mrs. Cohen, what on earth is the matter with you? Stop crying. I think your wife is DEPRESSED!"

"Yeah."

"This is not satisfactory. Depression is very BAD for this baby. Melina, this mother has the worst case of postpartum depression I have ever seen. Don't you think so?"

"Yes, I agree with you, Abigail, she seems to be very depressed."

"Listen up, Mrs. Cohen, I am writing a memo to your gynecologist right now . . . 'Mrs. Cohen has the WORST case of POSTPARTUM DEPRESSION I have ever seen. She MUST see a PSYCHIATRIST who specializes in postpartum. RIGHT AWAY, before she does damage to herself or her baby. Please make psychiatric REFERRAL for Mrs. Cohen. My recommendation would be Dr. Bellucci, who specializes in POSTPARTUM depression. Yours truly, Abigail Arbogast.' 'Call the adoption agency'—that's the most ridiculous thing I ever heard. Never heard a mother say a thing like that before. Did you ever hear a mother say a thing like that, Melina?"

"No, Abigail, I did not."

"Dad, make sure your wife sees a psychiatrist right away. And come back in a month. I want to monitor this baby very, very carefully. You'll bring her back next month. You are very, very lucky that I am seeing Elayna from such a young age."

* * *

Dr. Levin referred us to a geneticist, who confirmed the diagnosis of Russell-Silver syndrome. "RSS is a rare growth disorder, with genetic causes that are complex and not well understood. In Eliana's case, Alice's advanced maternal age may have played a part, but it's impossible to determine."

We brought Eliana to the pediatric orthopedic surgeon whom Levin praised as "the best in the field, as well as the nicest guy you'd ever hope to meet." Dr. Melody's patients looked nothing like the children in Levin's waiting room, whom I'd envied for their perfect symmetry. The crowded hospital clinic waiting room looked like a war zone, strewn with miniature, injured soldiers; babies whose spines and faces were contorted in pain; a big kid sitting immobile in an electric wheelchair fitted with a back brace and oxygen tank; children missing limbs, or with limbs so mismatched it seemed impossible that they belonged to the same body; a toddler whose enormous head was too heavy for her neck to support unassisted. Michael and I looked up at the same time to see a family wheel in a child who was so grotesquely deformed she or he did not look quite human. More a Frankenstein-like assemblage of mismatched parts, ripped apart and crudely resewn, features splattered onto its face in angry disorder. Boy? Girl? Age? It was impossible to tell. The child's toddler sister played quietly on the floor beside the wheelchair with two Barbie dolls. The parents looked tired. It was difficult not to stare.

So we looked at Eliana, who was peacefully lying in my lap, playing with Michael's fingers. We looked at her perfect rosebud lips. Rosy cheeks. Alert and sparkling blue green eyes. Soft, glowing skin. She kicked her legs. She grabbed Michael's hand and sucked on his finger. She made eager baby sounds.

She looked beautiful and complete and content.

"She's a good candidate for leg-lengthening surgery," said Dr. Melody, gently holding Eliana, making eye contact with her as he bent her knees and circled her legs to test her flexibility. "If Eliana's leg-length discrepancy remains proportional to her overall size, at full height her right leg will be about five inches shorter than her left leg. In early childhood, a shoe lift will suffice, but I predict that she'll need at least two lengthening surgeries, one on the tibia and one on the femur."

"How do you lengthen a leg?" asked Michael.

"Luckily, bone grows. Broken bones regenerate. So we cut the bone in half . . ."

Michael looked as if he might faint. I squeezed his cold, damp hand with my cold, damp hand.

". . . and we stabilize the leg with an external frame. Then we literally turn a screw every day for about two months, to separate and lengthen the severed bone—it's called 'bone distraction.' Each day a tiny amount of new bone fills in the gap."

"Does it hurt?" I asked.

"Yes, it does. It's not just the bone that has to lengthen. We're stretching the soft tissue and muscles and ligaments and nerves, which can be quite painful. Sometimes we have to do additional surgeries to cut and lengthen the soft tissue. It takes up to a year to fully recuperate."

Now I feel like fainting.

"But kids are pretty resilient. I expect that Eliana will spend two years of her childhood going through this. It's no fun, but without leg-lengthening, she'll probably have chronic back pain as an adult, and wearing a five-inch shoe lift is not a good thing. Let's wait and see. There may be some catch-up growth in the right leg as she gets older.

"Bring Eliana back in six months. I want to keep a close watch on her scoliosis. Perhaps her physical therapist can straighten this C-curve. Otherwise, we might consider back surgery."

Wrongful Life

"You have a strong case. I'll take it on," said Joan Miller, the medical malpractice lawyer I'd spoken to during my pregnancy. "I'm personally interested in pushing the envelope on these cases if I possibly can. But, Alice, are you up to this? It's hell going through a lawsuit, I guarantee you. You'll have to say things under oath that Eliana might ultimately have access to, so you have to think about that too. And I'm no picnic for my clients, you should know that. I'm going to be very, very tough on you; you're going to have to work very hard on this case. And it could take three years for the case to go to trial. Do you have any questions?"

"Is it a problem that we can't prove Russell-Silver syndrome was caused by the medical malpractice?"

"Not at all. You just have to prove that there was malpractice— a no-brainer in this case, since your gynecologist was a moron! A total fucking moron! Pardon my French. I can't believe she did an internal exam when you were five months pregnant and told you—what? That you had a bladder problem? Loss of muscle tone? She shouldn't be allowed to practice medicine.

"You have what's called a 'wrongful life' case. Are you familiar with the term?"

"No."

"'Wrongful life' refers to a class of legal cases in which the birth itself is a result of the malpractice. That's what you're saying—isn't it? That you wouldn't have had this baby if it weren't for your doctors' mistakes? Wrongful life is controversial, because it implies that a child shouldn't have been born. Ultimately, it's predicated on a prochoice position. It gets into ethical gray areas. It's political. Juries and judges don't want to go on record saying that a particular child should not have been born. Most lawyers quite frankly don't like to touch 'wrongful life' cases with a ten-foot pole."

"You're very, very limited in what you can sue for. Damages are limited to the additional and extraordinary expenses of raising a child with special needs. You can't sue for the ordinary expenses of childrearing, and you can't sue for emotional injury. The legal precedent is very clear. If the child is healthy, even if the birth was a result of unmistakable medical malpractice, you can't sue. Period. You only have a case if the baby has a sickness or disability, which will result in expenses over and above the cost of raising a healthy child. If you, the mother, suffered emotional injury as a result of the medical malpractice, you can't sue for that. If your child suffers emotional injury as a result of the medical malpractice, you can't sue for that. Even if the mother is impoverished, you can't sue for the cost of food and shelter for an unexpected, unbidden child.

"Bottom line, the court presumes that having a child is a good thing, that life is a good thing. The legal precedent in 'wrongful life' cases is very clear, but I want to push the envelope. I'm an extremely aggressive prosecutor. This is a feminist issue, and I'd like to take this on. There's no financial risk for you. In med-mal cases, the client pays nothing unless the case is won or settled in your favor, in which case the lawyer gets thirty percent and the client gets seventy percent. Let me know what you decide."

Michael wants nothing, nothing, absolutely nothing to do with the case. He doesn't believe in the premise of "wrongful life."

"Go ahead, Alice, have your lawsuit. Good luck. I hope you win a lot of money. I hope you and Eliana don't get hurt in the process. Just don't talk to me about it. I'm not part of this lawsuit, so keep my name out of it. I wish we could just get on with our lives as a family instead of dwelling on what's over, on what might have been."

"We're going into debt, Michael. We can't afford to pay for our crappy insurance, much less the doctors Eliana sees every week."

"We're not a family with one 'wrongful life.' "

"Growth hormone costs $15,000 a year. Who knows what the surgeries will cost?"

"We're not four people, three of whom were meant to be born and one who wasn't."

"If I win this case, her surgeries and doctors' visits and medication and who knows what else will be paid for. Do the math, Michael. I have to do this for Eliana."

"I don't want anything to do with this lawsuit."

* * *

We are, meanwhile, paying the minimum fees on our mounting credit card bills. I'm editing *Play by Play*, but I can't tour, so my income is minimal. Michael is touring—school shows in upstate New York, corporate performances in Chicago for Arthur Andersen. He's flying around the country. We're both taking on as much work as we can.

I hire a babysitter so I can get my work done. Jasmine the babysitter charges a lot because she has to pay a babysitter to take care of her daughter in Brooklyn while she's babysitting Eliana in Manhattan. Eliana is expensive. We go deeper into debt.

I sign a contract with Joan Miller and sign dozens of release forms so that she can gather evidence. My lawsuit on Eliana's behalf gives me a sense of maternal purpose. I'm getting really good at the advocacy part of parenting: like finding a doctor for Eliana when every doctor has said no; like taping tubes to my nipples so Eliana will be fortified by my meager allotment of breast milk; like suing for medical malpractice.

My mother the sociology professor taught me, "The way to change people's attitudes is to first change their behavior. Their attitudes will follow." I trust my mother's faith in this tenet of social science. If I can just master the behavior, make a habit of maternal self-sacrifice, the rest—

The rest? I can't remember what "the rest" is, just that there's something missing. What is it? I close my eyes and search for that thing I used to have. It glimmers briefly and eludes recognition. What am I looking for? A brilliance of light and color? An effortless sense of connection? An illogical perception of delight? Ecstatic yearning? A dimension of emotional texture and depth that I once took for granted but is now hidden, and if I could just remember what I'm looking for, I could remember where it's hidden? As a little kid, I used to think, "When I'm a mommy, I will do X and I won't do Y," keeping an inventory in my head of the things I would do just like my mother did, and the things I'd do differently when I had children, and now that I'm a mother who's forgotten how to be one, I wish I could remember the maternal manifesto I believed so adamantly when I was six, I could really use it, but the X and Y details are lost, so I'll grab hold of whatever I can grab hold of, which is "If I can just master the behavior, make a habit of maternal self-sacrifice—"

—the rest (I hope) will follow.

Decisions

"You are severely depressed," says Dr. Bellucci, the psychiatrist Dr. Arbogast insisted I see. She specializes in postpartum depression and other disorders related to childbirth. "I'm going to prescribe an antidepressant."

"No. Antidepressants are absorbed by breast milk. I exposed Eliana to enough chemicals before she was born. I don't want to inflict on her the unknown secondary effects of the serotonin reuptake inhibitor you want me to take."

"Would you consider stopping nursing and getting treatment for your depression so that you can bond properly with Eliana?"

"I'm nursing her till she's six months old."

"You told me she's not getting much breast milk."

"She's getting *some*. And I feel *very* bonded to her. I didn't for a while, but this is who I am now. I've given up everything else for her."

"You also told me you fantasize about throwing yourself in front of a moving truck, which I'm sure you agree would be very harmful to Eliana."

"I'm not really going to kill myself, I just imagine it. And it's usually not when I'm with Eliana. It's only when I'm alone that I get hit with these ninety-five-mile-an-hour hardball pitches into my brain, with these terrible, suicidal fantasies."

"I can prescribe meds proven to have the lowest absorption rate by breast milk. You can take it just before Eliana goes to sleep so it will be out of the breast milk before you nurse her. Here, you can read the studies."

I tried two different antidepressants.

Zoloft made me feel temporarily psychotic. In the middle of a sleepless night, my mind raced, and I was overwhelmed with waking nightmares. Paxil had the opposite effect. It took two weeks for anything to happen. Then I was slightly sedated, physically relaxed if a bit groggy. The suicidal thoughts ended.

"It takes the edge off your depression, doesn't it?" asked Dr. Bellucci.

Can you take the edge off something with no edge? Depression has an amorphous shape, no edges or corners, an all-encompassing cloud. My depression itself, the debilitating sense of hopelessness, was a dulling experience. At its worst the dullness made me feel poisoned. Paxil filtered out the poison. I was able to sleep through the night. "Yes, it takes the edge off."

Smiling

Eliana started smiling.

So did I.

It's heaven when your baby smiles at you. It causes mothers and fathers to fall in love, over and over, every time she smiles.

She started to read at six weeks.

Okay, that's the inflated claim of a doting mother. She wasn't reading, but she was fascinated by books. And I swear, when she was six weeks old I read *Goodnight Moon* to her, and when I said, "Turn the page, Eliana," she jerked her tiny hand to the cardboard page and pushed it to the left. Every page!

At the end of January, I got my period, the only time in fifteen years I'd had a period while not on ERT.

"Good lord, Alice, you certainly are not low-estrogen anymore, if you ever were," said Barbara, now my regular gynecologist. "Very few women get their periods so soon after giving birth. Your reproductive system is on go, that's for sure. You'll definitely have to use birth control if you don't want to get pregnant again."

Scene 4

Home Remedies

Eliana's Early Intervention home services begin in February.

Cathy, the physical therapist, comes to our apartment three mornings a week. She asks me to be in the room with them for the whole hour. She could use the extra set of hands. I hold Eliana's ankles while Cathy stretches her over a therapy ball to straighten her C-curve. It hurts her to be stretched like this and she cries every time, which makes me cry. But Cathy is an inspiring coach. She talks Eliana through the process, encouraging her all the while she is crying. Then, as soon as each stretching session is over, Cathy holds her, and Eliana is all smiles and hugs. Despite the pain she associates with Cathy's visits, the moment Cathy shows up at the apartment Eliana smiles and squeals with excitement.

Cathy improvises like an artist. She used to be a dancer, and she's translated her creative passions into her Early Intervention work. She scopes out the apartment for props, turns a pillow, a teddy bear, and a cereal box into an obstacle course.

Sometimes Cathy shows up with her two-year-old son,

Todd—"Hope you don't mind. This is totally against Early Intervention rules, but my babysitter didn't show"—and the session turns into a work session cum play date, toddler and infant equally curious about each other. Cathy assigns Todd jobs that make him feel important, like shaking bells and rattles to cheer Eliana up after she's been stretched.

One day Eliana and I show off to Cathy how she's learning to hold my hands to pull herself up to standing, and Cathy goes ballistic. "Don't you dare let her walk before she crawls," she admonishes me, as if I'd let Eliana put her hand in fire, "or her proprioceptive responses will never develop properly!"

"Her what?"

"Proprioceptive senses are sensory nerve terminals in the muscles, tendons, and joints that keep track of your body position and movement. Proprioception tells the brain about the position of your body parts in relation to one another, and the position of your body in relation to the world."

"Why is crawling important?"

"The infant develops proprioceptive responses through her knees and her toes and her hands when she crawls. It has to happen in infancy, or forget about it. Caput. Window of opportunity closed. Hey, Eliana, ya hear what I told your mom? Don't think you can wheedle out of crawling, just 'cause you're cute. It doesn't have to be pretty, but you have to get around on all fours before you walk. Capeesh?

"Because of Eliana's asymmetry, it's super important for her to learn how to walk on any surface: level or uneven; barefoot or wearing shoes; with or without a shoe lift; with or without leg-lengthening. Her proprioception has to be more versatile than other kids. She has to be like a proprioceptive genius! So, like, when she's a toddler, she can get out of bed barefoot and not fall down; and when she's ten and she's at the beach body surfing, and a wave knocks her down, she'll be able to stand up and get her balance even with the shifting sands and the undertow; and when she's twenty or fifty or eighty, and she's dancing with her lover or she's climbing a mountain, her proprioceptive nerves will automatically compensate for changes in level in the surface below her feet; changes in the height of the shoe lift she's wearing; changes in her leg length if she has surgery."

I love picturing Eliana body surfing, dancing with her lover, climbing a mountain. I love Cathy for permanently replacing the "we don't know if she'll ever walk" picture with these "she can do anything" pictures.

Once baby Eliana persuades Cathy of her commitment to crawling—executed with an unorthodox pattern of knees, elbows, hands, and toes—Cathy permits her to stand upright, with our assistance. Cathy raids Eliana's toy box and randomly arranges a colorful set of cardboard stacking cubes in a circle of large and small boxes. She holds Eliana up by her waist, I hold her hands, and she points her teeny toes and steps from one cube to another. Up-down. Up-up. Down-down. Higher-lower. Longer leg down—shorter leg even lower. Bigger foot up—smaller foot higher. Longer leg *way* up—then *way* down with the shorter leg.

Eliana laughs, amused by the surprising changes in elevation in the homemade amusement park ride on her bedroom floor. Her baby-voiced laughter is infectious; laughter begets laughter. Eliana's open-mouthed giggles, released by each delighted up-down astonishment, make me laugh so hard I'm gasping for breath, which makes Eliana laugh even more, which makes me nearly fall over, which makes Eliana gigglier and her cheeks rosier as she opens her mouth wide to let out each next peal of laughter.

"Her proprioceptive senses are having a field day!" says Cathy, her PT juices flowing. "Think of all the information she's absorbing through the soles of her feet."

Brynna, the oral-motor-speech therapist, comes once a week, with a box of bubblegum-flavored rubber surgical gloves for poking around inside Eliana's mouth. She wants complete privacy in her sessions. Behind Eliana's closed door, I hear Brynna sing. Eliana smiles at Brynna when she arrives, so I figure it's going well.

Joanna, the occupational therapist, starts two months after the other two therapists; I guess babies don't need help with their occupations till they're four months old. I can't decipher the language of OT. When Joanna waves her magic wand, she wishes for "normalization of tone in shoulder girdle, encouraging greater trunk stability, rotational integration of postural reactions as well as greater integration of tactile, vestibular, and proprioceptive experiences."

"Can I help during your sessions?" I ask.

"No. But I want you to brush her with a mushroom brush every day. Brush her whole body for five minutes every morning and every evening. Brush in long vertical strokes, from top to bottom. Cover every inch of her skin, and never brush the same place twice. Always brush her at the same time of day, except for the two days a week that I see her, when I will brush her myself. Any questions?"

"What's a mushroom brush?"

"You don't know? It's the soft, plastic brush you use to brush dirt off mushrooms."

"Oh!" I guess I've been too rough on my mushrooms all these years. "Why are we brushing her with a mushroom brush?"

"A brushing program is very effective for sensory integration, especially with high-tone babies like Eliana."

Joanna gives us a supply of yellow plastic mushroom brushes and we get with the program. Michael, Julia, and I take turns brushing naked Ellie—Julia has successfully initiated "Ellie" as an occasional nickname, with variations including "El," "Elbow," and Julia's personal favorite, "Elbow Macaroni."

"High-tone," "sensory integration," and "proprioception" slip into our everyday vocabulary, though Michael and I don't completely understand why we're brushing our baby like a delicate mushroom twice a day.

But Eliana enjoys being brushed, we like brushing her, and she lights up whenever she sees Joanna . . . and Cathy . . . and Brynna, who in my unprofessional opinion are all geniuses.

Even Dr. Abigail Arbogast gets smiles from Eliana, though she leaves us in the waiting room for ages before every appointment. Dr. Arbogast is fiercely dedicated to her Russell-Silver syndrome patients, and she will do everything in her power to help Eliana thrive and grow.

Scene 5

April Fools

In early March, Dani Athena called. I hadn't seen her since my fall semester solo theater class. I'd been thinking about her, wondering if she was still alive.

"I'm having an April Fools party and I want you to come. You'll have a wonderful time, and it would mean a lot to me if you were there."

"I'd love to come. . . . How are you?"

"Terrible. The cancer has spread all over. I've decided against chemo treatment because it would add only a few months, if that much. Anyway, I want to have this party. It will be a performance . . . the next incarnation of the piece I started in your class."

Dani's April Fools party was in her friend's loft in Tribeca. Lit by dozens of candles, the maple floors glowed, the room shimmered and gave everybody the look of a hand-painted antique photo, rosy cheeks and red lips over sepia skin. Dani was much thinner than when I'd last seen her. Her sleeveless silk dress bared her angular collarbone and neck. Her guests were feasting on a buffet of Greek food.

Dani handed each new guest a playing card and instructed us to find the other person at the party who had the same card. This party game ensured that her disparate guests introduced themselves to one another and shared stories, talked about how they knew Dani, and ate and drank with one another in their quest for their card's mate. I found the mate to my eight of hearts, Katrina, a dance teacher who taught with Dani. Katrina and I sat down with our paper plates of moussaka and stuffed grape leaves and plastic cups of red wine.

Many of Dani's guests were dancers, some of them teenagers, several elderly white-haired dancers, and a little boy in tights and ballet shoes. The dancers darted and disappeared barefoot into hidden rooms and sleeping lofts, followed by the resident golden retriever, and reemerged in costumes, carrying props and musical instruments.

A pair of high school students in brightly colored sashes ushered everybody to the designated performance space, folding chairs facing a wall draped with Indian fabrics. Dani sat crosslegged on the floor, holding a single playing card—the Joker—and facing the audience. The room quieted. We looked at Dani. She looked at us, her skeletal body very still under the flickering candlelight, her dark eyes ablaze, deeply inhaling the room full of friends and students and teachers and dancers and poets and musicians and admirers. Only the muffled sound of traffic from seven floors below, a clock ticking, the dog's tail rhythmically slapping the floor, and the sound of Dani's breathing. There was a tacit understanding in the room of the implications of this silent exchange—Dani was saying good-bye, celebrating her life, welcoming her death, asking us to remember her.

After several minutes, she bowed to us and took a seat in the audience. A ragtag performance ensued. Kids and old folks bumped into one another, leaping onto the stage whenever there was a lull. The performance boundaries dissolved, tricksters and clowns emerged from every corner. An old man played a balalaika on top of the refrigerator. A young woman recited Hamlet's soliloquy from inside a clothes hamper. Teenagers read their poems aloud in the bathroom. Nearly everybody took a turn—played the recorder, danced, recited from Ovid and from *The Brady Bunch*, sang Beatles songs and Irish ballads and Greek folk songs. At midnight, Dani gathered us again. Her face was flushed with sickness and euphoria. "It's late, but for anybody who can stay, my wonderful friends Pablo and Conchita will teach you how to tango."

Men and women, men and men, women and girls, the little boy and the dog, paired up to tango. I couldn't stay. Michael was flying to Chicago early the next morning and I'd promised not to be back too late. I said good-bye to Dani. "Tonight I found the way to tell the story I needed to tell!" she said. I hugged her, running my fingertips over her bare back, feeling the outline of every vertebra and rib. On the street, I looked up at the candlelit windows on the seventh floor.

She died in May.

Solo Theater

I told my solo theater class about Dani's April Fools party—the event as the culminating performance of her life, her performance as a gift, her discovery of the story she wanted to tell and how she wanted to tell it, the connectedness of performance and ritual, clowning and death. My students indulged me by listening politely, though they were less interested in Dani's story than in their own. They were fairly bursting to get back to their own stories of first love.

It was Ken's turn to perform. He asked if someone would read the voice-over for his new scene while he danced and mimed the story. Esther Levine volunteered. He handed her his script, and Esther read with total commitment and not a hint of self-consciousness, endowing his text with her squeaky, eighty-four-year-old Brooklyn-inflected voice: "When we were hidden in the darkness in Central Park, Enrico asked me to unzip him. I pulled down his jeans and I saw the biggest cock I'd ever seen in my entire life. I put my mouth on his huge dick, while cradling his enormous balls in my hand. He pushed my head down on him over and over. . . ."

After the class gave Ken feedback on his new scene, it was Esther's turn to perform her piece. She had been writing a play about her long marriage. For four decades, she had silently submitted to her husband's verbal abuse and sexual infidelities. Each week, she presented a new scene from her marriage, in reverse order, from the end of her marriage to the beginning. The effect was of Esther getting younger each week. Early in the semester she performed the last scene of her marriage, when she walked out on her husband in 1972 in an unprecedented act of feminist rage. Tonight she performed the first scene of her play—her wedding night in the summer of 1940.

In our fluorescent-lit classroom, Esther shed sixty years to channel her twenty-four-year-old self in a room in the Plaza

Hotel. "Ah, ah, ah, ahh, ahhh, aaahhh, aaaah, aaaaahhhh, AAAAAHHH, AAAAAAHHHHH, AAAAAAAA!!!!!! . . . ahh-hhhhh, aaa . . ."

Esther arched her ancient back on the folding metal chair, her body shuddering as she relished her first orgasm with her husband. She sighed loudly and slowly, allowed the soft wrinkled folds of her body to sink sensuously into her chair. "Oh, Jerome, I'm so relaxed. Shall we go to Ruby Foo's for Chinese?"

Scene 6

The Wedding

"Are we really having a wedding in June?" asked Michael reasonably in mid-April.

"I guess so. We already paid for it, didn't we?"

"Don't we have to do things? Like invite people?"

Because we had no time, we planned in no time. We made and printed our own invitations, "Michael, Alice, Julia, and Eliana invite you to celebrate our wedding and our new family." Julia punched holes in the cards and tied silver ribbons through them. We all stuffed envelopes. We invited everybody we knew, hoping not to exceed our space and budget limit of one hundred, and predicted accurately that few of our out-of-town friends and relatives would come.

I phoned the French chef at Round Hill House, chose a menu—interesting food for the grown-ups, boring food, at Julia's request, for the kids. I asked if he could also take care of the flowers, on our minimal budget.

"You are zee bride. What type of flowers do you want?" he asked.

"Whatever you think looks best. You know more than I do about flowers."

"What are your colors? Zee bride always has strong opinions about flowers."

"Not me. I trust you completely," I said, holding the receiver with my chin, retaping the formula tube to my nipple after spilling formula on Eliana's head, and feeling exceptionally unbridelike.

We got our marriage license and hired Dan, an unorthodox cantor, to officiate at our decidedly unorthodox mixed marriage.

We booked a bus and driver to drive our car-free Manhattan friends to and from Round Hill House, an hour north of the city.

We enlisted Eliana's babysitter Jasmine to come with us.

I bought fluffy dresses for the girls. Michael rented a tux.

"Buy this pale gold dress, it looks great," said my friend Melissa, who pulled me from store to store on a high-speed shopping trip four days before my wedding. "Get these shoes. No, you don't have time to look in another shoe store. Buy these stockings. This bra. This lipstick. This necklace."

The night before the wedding, I packed the wedding essentials—our marriage license, Eliana's diapers, bottles of formula. Eliana was six months old, and she and I had amicably agreed to stop breastfeeding as scheduled. I dumped the plastic tubes and tape in the trash without a trace of nostalgia.

Round Hill was a gorgeous, big old house with a wraparound porch, reminiscent of a southern plantation.

"I hope you are happy with zee flowers I chose," said the French chef. He had bought roses of a breathtaking deep orange. I couldn't imagine more beautiful flowers.

It was an overcast morning. Our guests were outside enjoying hors d'oeuvres on Round Hill's beautiful grounds, when there was the rumble of thunder. Dan urged us to start the outdoor ceremony immediately.

The marriage license was not in the suitcase. It wasn't anywhere. More thunder. I panicked, but Dan calmly assured us, "When you sign the katubah"—the Jewish wedding contract we'd written ourselves—"you'll be married under Jewish law. New York State can wait till you find the license, and your guests don't have to know."

The gusty wind blew women's long hair and long dresses helter-skelter. Our friend Mark, Sophie's dad, played guitar. Michael and I walked hand in hand down the aisle and stood under the chuppah—the traditional Jewish wedding canopy, the corner poles held by my sisters, Michael's sister, and his best friend, Sean. My long skirt danced frenetically. The sky darkened to an ominous gray, the leaves flashed silver. A roll of thunder and a few drops of rain. Our guests squirmed anxiously in their folding chairs.

Dan began by teasing us. "In Jewish tradition, rain at a wedding signifies fertility." Michael and I groaned. Everybody laughed, except Eliana, who started to cry. Jasmine took Eliana from Julia's lap, and quieted her with a bottle. A moment later, the wind died down and a ray of sun lit the chuppah. Our guests applauded. The sun shone for the rest of the ceremony. Julia carried our wedding rings to us on a silk pillow, Michael's mother read a passage from the New Testament. We recited the Hebrew wedding prayer Dan had taught us, we exchanged rings, we kissed, we were married.

A clap of thunder. Everybody raced into the house and it poured for the rest of the day. At the end of the party, I led the Second Line, the traditional New Orleans jazz parade celebrated at weddings and funerals. Michael's mom and his sister and his aunts and his girl cousins and I held miniature decorative umbrellas, which bobbed up and down as we snaked and circled and zigzagged—our mixed-up, mismatched wedding rituals weaving our mixed-up, mismatched family together.

The owner of Round Hill House found our marriage license the next day under a bag of Pampers, behind a chair, where Jasmine had changed Eliana. We went to Dan's apartment to sign, my sisters and Michael's lesbian friends from high school joining us as witnesses. For our brief, euphoric honeymoon on Block Island—while Daisy stayed home with the girls—Michael and I crammed as much bike riding, lovemaking, and lobster-roll-feasting into three days as we possibly could.

Under the careful tutelage of her physical therapist, Eliana's body began to straighten out of the C-curve. She became stronger. Her tight muscles relaxed.

So did mine.

Eliana delighted in the new sights and sounds of summer.

So did I.

She smiled more.

So did I.

Life was good again.

Tuh! Tuh! Tuh!

What I Know

I love both my daughters.

The one who was planned for, researched, fought for, hard-won, rehearsed for, competed for, and paid for on the not-for-profit Spence-Chapin adoption agency's sliding scale.

I love the one who arrived unannounced and impossibly.

I love the one who was adopted, whose birth I observed from a comfortable and pain-free distance.

I love the one I gave birth to at age forty-five, after forty-seven awful hours of labor.

I love the one whose birth mother didn't know about her until she was six months pregnant.

I love the one I didn't know about, until I was six months pregnant.

I love the one who is off-the-charts tall and the one who's off-the-charts short.

I love the dark-haired one and the fair-haired one.

I love the symmetrical one and the asymmetrical one.

I love the one I desperately wanted, and the one I desperately didn't want.

The Bat Mitzvah and the Trial

Three years later. Julia is thirteen. Eliana is almost four.

Julia's bat mitzvah rehearsal was on a Wednesday afternoon, November 8, 2003, ten days before her bat mitzvah—the Jewish rite of passage for a thirteen-year-old girl. Standing between the rabbi and the cantor, taller than the rabbi and looking very grown up, Julia chanted confidently from the Torah in Hebrew, despite her bad cold, while Michael and I cheered her on from the otherwise empty synagogue. Eliana was having too good a time running through the aisles to pay attention to Julia's run-through.

November 8 was also the day before my medical malpractice trial was to begin. Originally scheduled for September, the defendant had twice requested a postponement, and the trial—expected to last for two weeks—now coincided uncomfortably with Julia's bat mitzvah.

Joan Miller, my lawyer, accurately predicted when Eliana was a newborn that the case would take at least three years to come to trial. Most of the trial preparation over those three-and-a-half years happened without my involvement. Joan periodically called me with questions, or asked me to come in to her midtown office to sign dozens of release forms. Two summers ago, she and I spent long hours preparing for three grueling days of deposition. The pretty, blond court stenographer typed three hundred pages of my testimony and cried through the emotional parts, while the defense lawyer grilled me and Joan kicked me under the table whenever I hesitated on a date or sequence of events. The defense attempted several times to have the case dismissed, for bogus reasons. Joan moved aggressively forward, welcoming a fight. Jury selection was complete. She assured me that tomorrow was the real deal.

Julia's Torah portion was Abraham's sacrifice of Isaac. When she finished the Hebrew chanting, she launched into the speech she'd written, a critique of Abraham's irresponsible parenting and of the political consequences of religious fanaticism.

"Why would Abraham do it? Why would he attempt to kill his son on God's command, without ever asking God why? How could you sacrifice your son? If you think about these people as real people, rather than just characters in a story, Abraham would probably later be filled with guilt, and Isaac would be terrified. If I had been Isaac, I wouldn't have been able to forgive my father for attempting to kill me, even if he said God commanded it. . . ."

While Julia calmly read her speech, Michael chased Eliana. She was so tiny and agile that he genuinely had trouble keeping up with her. She raced up and down the aisles, climbed onto my lap for a half second, then scooted through the empty rows of velvet-cushioned chairs and initiated an unauthorized game of hide-and-seek. Michael tried to entertain Eliana without disrupting the rehearsal, which he assessed by the number of times the rabbi looked up at him with pursed lips.

"Today, I think it's really important to question what people say are God's commandments. When the Spanish took over Central and South America, killing thousands of people, they did it in God's name. When suicide bombers recently attacked in Israel, they did it in God's name. When the Crusaders slaughtered thousands of people, they did it in God's name. When the Spanish Inquisition persecuted Jews and Protestants and Muslims, they did it in God's name. . . ."

Eliana wore a short, blue dress over purple sweatpants and red canvas lace-up sneakers, the right sneaker, the one with the shoe lift, two sizes smaller than the left one. She was little enough to squeeze under the auditorium seats, and she kept disappearing and reappearing several rows away, her wavy mop of golden brown hair briefly popping into view, her beautiful blue green eyes ablaze, her red-cheeked face lighting up with a smile and a squeal of pleasure when she caught sight of Michael, before vanishing under the seats again.

"When terrorists attacked the Twin Towers on 9/11, they did it in God's name. When George Bush invaded Iraq, he said it was his religious responsibility—he did it in God's name. Maybe if these people had actually stopped and thought about what they were being ordered to do, the world would be a better place. . . ."

Eliana's dress was dustier each time she emerged from under the seats. Michael finally caught her and carried her upstairs to the playroom, when he decided that Eliana's giggly game was trying the patience even of Julia, who was valiantly sneezing through the end of her speech.

Eliana was enrolled in the synagogue's preschool upstairs. Her teachers reported that she didn't interact much with the other children and spent a lot of time playing alone in the sandbox. Eliana reported that she loved playing alone in the sandbox but that she was tired of the children pointing at her shoe lift every day and asking, "Why do you have a big shoe?" and, "Why are you so little? You look like a baby." I tried to make play dates for her with her classmates but met with little success. The preschool director was strongly urging us to keep Eliana in preschool for an additional year, to develop her social skills. She'd be just old enough to start kindergarten at the local public school next fall, but with her December birthday she'd be the youngest in the class. Michael and I weren't sure she'd be ready for kindergarten, nor were we convinced that this preschool was an environment where her social skills would flourish. We mulled and fretted and wondered how we'd ever decide, until Julia-the-Straightforward cut to the chase and asked her little sister, "Hey, Elbow, would you rather go to kindergarten at a new school next fall, or stay an extra year in preschool?

"I want to go to kindergarten at a new school!" Eliana shouted, without hesitation.

Just as Julia's rehearsal was ending, my cell phone rang. Michael took the girls home, while I sat in the empty synagogue for the next hour talking to my lawyer. Joan quizzed me on my testimony and yelled at me for my inconsistencies.

"Go home and reread the three-hundred-page transcript of your depositions. Make sure you memorize every word! Any inconsistency on the witness stand will throw your credibility into question and alienate the jury, if they're not already turned off by the premise of 'wrongful life.' This isn't going to be easy. Didn't I tell you to memorize that goddamn transcript weeks ago? I warned you that I was tough, didn't I?"

After dinner, Michael bathed Eliana and put her to bed while I rushed Julia through her homework and into her pajamas and then sat down sleepily in the living room to review the daunting transcript.

I paused to listen to Michael, who was in the bedroom, playing his guitar and singing. He'd been out of work for eighteen months to date. His unemployment benefits, which had been extended twice, were about to run out. The silver lining to this depressing scenario was that he had time to make music again.

When Eliana was a year old, Michael took a full-time job with Arthur Andersen—combining a desk job in internal communications with writing and performing for their training conferences and recruiting events, as he'd done for years. We joked that he performed corporate types so persuasively that they mistook him for the real thing. Michael's transition—from unpredictable freelance career to full-time job with benefits at one of the Big Five accounting firms—was the epitome of a safe move.

But a year after he took the job, Arthur Andersen was indicted by the Department of Justice on charges of obstruction of justice, for shredding documents related to its audit of Enron. Suddenly, mind-blowingly, the century-old accounting behemoth fell. Nearly twenty-eight thousand employees lost their jobs. In June 2002 the company was convicted, and Andersen was out of business.

In his unanticipated free time, Michael was working on two new solo shows: a children's play called *Beanstalk Jacques*, a Cajun retelling of *Jack and the Beanstalk* set in the Louisiana Bayou; and a one-man musical about the downfall of Arthur Andersen, called *Simple Addition: How I Brought Down a Global Accounting Firm*—a dark comedy about the seductive power of money and the place of individual responsibility within a huge corporation—a satirical retelling of what Michael believed to be, with twenty-twenty hindsight, his complicity in the Andersen debacle, the small part he played in facilitating the ethical compromises that led to the company's demise.

His new lyrics were really good. So was his guitar playing, which I hadn't heard for the year he was working at Andersen. I felt like the real Michael was back; supremely ethical, cynical, smart, funny, penniless (though this time not by choice) Michael was back. Unfortunately, there were bills to pay.

Since Andersen fell, we'd gone deeply into debt. Preschool in Manhattan was insanely expensive, as were Eliana's medical costs. My income was modest. Michael's was nil. I had to win this case for Eliana or we would never get out of debt.

It was nearly 10:30. I would have preferred to sleep, but I hoisted the unwieldy deposition transcript into my lap.

The phone rang.

"Hello, this is Juan-Carlos from Café Maya. How are you? Listen, Alice, I have very bad news. A building inspector came in today to check on a leak in the basement. It turns out the whole foundation is sinking into the earth, and they have to close the building until it's repaired. . . . I'm so sorry, but we cannot have Julia's bat mitzvah party here next Saturday. . . . No, not for months. . . . I know, I know, I feel terrible. . . . I was looking forward to wearing—what do you call it?—yes, a yamaca. . . . But listen, I will try to help you. I have a friend with a new tapas restaurant in the neighborhood. Maybe he can help us. Can you meet me outside the café in fifteen minutes?"

Julia's bat mitzvah is in one week, and we suddenly have no place for the party.

My trial for Eliana is tomorrow morning, and I have three hundred pages to memorize.

How do I prioritize tomorrow's court appearance on behalf of Eliana versus next week's bat mitzvah for Julia? The bat mitzvah, in addition to Julia's seven years of study and six months of intensive preparation, represents a year of research and planning, resulting in the small miracle of finding a restaurant that would have a party for seventy-five guests on our small budget. The outcome of Eliana's medical malpractice, three years in the works, will impact Eliana's access to medical care and our family's quality of life.

"Julia, wake up and get dressed. I know you just went to bed, but we're going out."

It was drizzling when we met Juan-Carlos outside Café Maya. It looked so inviting through the windows, with its deep red walls and a little upstairs party space just large enough for Julia and her friends. A sign on the door read, CLOSED BY ORDER OF NYC DEPARTMENT OF BUILDINGS. Black-haired, elegant Juan-Carlos kissed me and Julia on both cheeks. "Come, my friend is expecting us."

We walked five blocks south on dark, rainy Columbus Avenue to a brand new tapas restaurant, an attractive, narrow café with a long wooden bar on one side, facing an intimate cluster of round wooden tables and chairs with mosaic tile seats. Pedro, the slender, sandy-haired proprietor, greeted Juan-Carlos with kisses on both cheeks.

"Pedro, this is my friend Alice and her daughter Julia. Julia is going to have her bat mitzvah next week, and they need a place for their party. Seventy-five people. Can you do it for them?"

"Sit, sit," Pedro instructed us. His easy smile made me want his restaurant to work out. Pedro whispered something to a waiter. In a moment there was a glass of sangria for me and a 7-Up for Julia, and a few small plates of fish, sausages, baby eels, sautéed peppers. Twenty-two customers comfortably filled the intimate restaurant.

"We can do this for you," said Pedro with bravura.

Julia whispered in my ear, "Mom, it's too small!"

"Um, Pedro, how will you fit seventy-five people?" I asked.

"Easy," said Pedro. He counted additional tables and chairs, currently in storage, and described a seating arrangement for seventy-five that, notwithstanding his confident tone, was 90 percent imagination. My skepticism was trumped by Julia's tears.

"It's too small," she whimpered.

"You're right, Julia," said Pedro thoughtfully. "I have a good friend in the neighborhood with a Turkish restaurant. He might help us out."

Pedro, Juan-Carlos, Julia, and I walked four more blocks in the rain, till we got to a Turkish restaurant on a side street just east of Columbus. When we opened the door we were greeted by sweet smells of coriander and cumin. Behind the antique wooden bar were blue-tiled walls, copper pots, a seating area with luxurious chairs upholstered in Middle Eastern tapestries of orange and gold. This was more upscale than Juan-Carlos's or Pedro's restaurant. This was way out of my budget.

Mahmood came to the door, a tall, commanding man with dark eyes and olive skin. Arms crossed over his chest, he allowed the more demonstrative Pedro and Juan-Carlos to exchange kisses with him on both cheeks. "What can I do for you?" he asked his fellow neighborhood restaurateurs, glancing at the sleepy, soggy thirteen-year-old and her bedraggled mother, whom his colleagues had dragged in from the rain. The fate of Julia's bat mitzvah was in the hands of these three men.

To persuade Mahmood, Juan-Carlos artfully painted his relationship with me as an enduring friendship, Pedro described Julia's upcoming bat mitzvah as a rite of passage of epic proportions and the matter of Juan-Carlos's sinking restaurant as a cataclysmic event. They took turns embellishing the story while they argued my case to Mahmood.

"I made the mother a promise a year ago."

"A Jewish girl's most important day."

"My restaurant is sinking into the very bowels of the earth."

"They have relatives coming from all over the world."

"I signed a contract with the mother."

"The mother is honest and honorable."

"She is not a rich woman."

"The girl has prepared for this ceremony her whole life."

"It is the day a girl becomes a woman."

"Julia's grandparents are traveling from Israel for the occasion."

Where did he get this? I have no relatives in Israel. A few guests were flying in from LA and New Orleans, but the rest were local. I kept my mouth shut while they spun their tall tale, my tall tale. The highly impassioned appeal by our rescuers was making an impression. Mahmood listened to his colleagues and then silently considered.

"I will honor the woman's contract. Your party will be here."

Julia shot me a panicked look, which meant, "Mom! I haven't even seen the restaurant yet, and isn't this my party? Does Mahmood even know how to make bland, teen-friendly food like hamburgers and French fries?" I signaled her with the slightest lift of my eyebrows to keep her mouth shut. She made a less subtle exasperated face at me, pursing her lips and gesturing with her thick eyebrows.

"Thank you very much, Mahmood. May I ask you a few questions?"

Now Pedro and Juan-Carlos made urgent eyebrow gestures at me, which meant, "Don't look a gift horse in the mouth!" and, "Let's go while the going's good." I tried to suppress my Jewish-mother-preparing-for-her-daughter's-bat-mitzvah instincts but couldn't suppress it entirely. I am, after all, a Jewish mother.

"Could we take a quick look at the restaurant?"

Mahmood's jaw muscles twitched, his left eyebrow raised slightly, but he led us into a beautiful octagonal dining room, which seated at least eighty.

"Barbara Walters is having her Christmas party here," he boasted.

Barbara Walters could afford a party here, but I was quite certain I could not.

"Oh, it's beautiful. Two more things. Could we talk about costs?"

Mahmood's jaw muscles twitched again. "Did you not hear me? I will honor your contract."

"Thank you!" I could hardly believe a party at this elegant

restaurant wouldn't cost more than a party at humble Café Maya. "And could you show us the menu?"

Mahmood's jaw twitched again. Juan-Carlos and Pedro looked exasperated.

"Don't worry. I will take care of everything."

Urgent whisper from Julia into my ear: "Ask him if they have hamburgers." I stepped on Julia's foot and slowly applied pressure while I shook Mahmood's hand.

"Thank you so much. I, thank you, I really appreciate . . ."

Pedro and Juan-Carlos were kissing Mahmood's cheeks and ushering me and Julia out the door as quickly as possible, before we blew it.

"Don't worry. Mahmood will take care of everything." My new mantra.

Julia and I walked back home in the rain. She quickly fell asleep. Michael was still playing guitar. I sat down to reread the deposition but couldn't keep my eyes open and decided it was futile anyway. I was never good at memorizing lines, but I remembered everything that happened, and would tell the story truthfully. I would leave it to my lawyer to artfully frame the truth in her dramatic retelling of my real-life tall tale. Like my restaurant allies tonight, I could count on her highly impassioned appeal to make the desired impression. My lawyer will take care of everything that Mahmood doesn't take care of.

I had erotic dreams that night about the three handsome restaurant owners, telling elaborate stories while they made love to me at once, mingling the flavors and scents of Mexican, Spanish, and Turkish food. I dreamed that Juan-Carlos was my lawyer and Mahmood was the judge and that Eliana was already a thirteen-year-old, healthy and robust and full-grown and confident and about to become a woman.

The next morning at City Hall I waited with my lawyer's associate outside the courtroom. Joan came out and whispered to me that the jury was ready to begin, but she was trying to negotiate a last-minute deal with the defending lawyer in the judge's chambers. I sat on the wooden bench outside the courtroom for two hours, with instructions not to say anything to anybody but to smile politely at everyone.

Joan had lined up two expert witnesses to speak on Eliana's behalf. Endocrinologist Dr. Abigail Arbogast, expert on Russell-Silver syndrome, has closely monitored Eliana since she was an infant and has protected her from Russell-Silver's most dangerous symptoms. Now she was chomping at the bit to share her expertise about Eliana's growth disorder to a captive audience of judge and jury. Eliana's more sedate orthopedic surgeon, Dr. Melody, has prepared a PowerPoint presentation, with compelling charts and graphs; X-rays of Eliana's legs; a slide show illustrating the multiple, complex surgeries Eliana was likely to need to correct her asymmetry; and a summary of her anticipated, astronomical medical expenses, every bit as scary as the graphics. Drs. Arbogast and Melody were scheduled to appear in court tomorrow. Today I would be the one on the witness stand.

Joan came out of the judge's chambers from time to time to give me whispered updates: "It's looking good." "It's not looking good." "I think we're about to settle." "They're not playing." "We're going to trial."

Midmorning, the jury was given a ten-minute break, and they glanced curiously at me as they exited the courtroom and walked down the echoing marble-floored hall. I smiled politely, per Joan's instructions, wondering what they thought of my "wrongful life" case. Joan hadn't told me a thing about the jury selection process. They reentered the courtroom and the hall was quiet again.

Once more, Joan came out and whispered to me, "They've made us an offer." She showed me the details of the offer. "Remember, in 'wrongful life' cases, damages are limited to the additional and extraordinary expenses of raising a child with special needs. If we go to trial—well, you never can tell with juries; they may be sympathetic, or they may hate the whole concept of 'wrongful life' and Eliana could end up with nothing. I think we should settle."

I agreed.

She whispered to me as she led me through the hall. "My only regret is that my expert witnesses never got to take the stand. They were going to be brilliant!"

Joan ushered me through the court, past the twelve bored-looking jury members and two alternates, and into the judge's chambers. Judge Snow, a stout woman in her sixties, moved about in her black robes with evident arthritic pain. But she smiled mischievously at me and shook my hand heartily when I thanked her on behalf of Eliana.

"This is not for vacations in Disneyland," she said, wagging her finger at me and knitting her thick eyebrows into one very persuasive eyebrow. "The purpose of this settlement is to make Eliana as healthy and strong as she possibly can be, do you understand?"

"I understand."

"Good! Now let's thank those jury members. They've been

sitting out there for two days. They must be bored to death. We'll give them this. I certainly don't need it," she said, lifting a large plastic bowl of Halloween candy from the table.

She limped out of her chambers to the courtroom with the bowl of Halloween candy.

"Ladies and gentlemen of the jury," she said, voice booming, face beaming. "We have arrived at a happy and fair settlement between both parties. The successful outcome of this litigation is due, in no small part, to your participation. Because you were out here, ready to serve, the two sides in there were motivated to come to an agreement. You have served well, the lawyers have served well, a sick child has been served well. Oh, and take some Halloween candy. As judge, I order you not to leave till the bowl is empty!"

To my surprise, the jury members lined up to meet me. I was a celebrity. Joan was a more potent storyteller than I'd given her credit for. The jury members liked me, sight unseen. They cared about Eliana. They knew that I wrote and performed for children. They were happy the case settled. They shook my hand and told me their own stories.

"My son got AIDS when he was thirty-five," said a frail, white-haired old woman, blue veins showing through translucent skin. "This was before AZT. He came back to live with me for his final months. At the end, I could barely recognize him, he was so thin, and covered with lesions. It's heartbreaking to see your child sick, at any age."

A young woman whispered, "When I was pregnant last summer, we found out the baby would have Down syndrome, so my husband and I decided to have an abortion. It was a painful decision, but I can't imagine not having that option. I think I would have gone crazy if I didn't have that choice."

"Hi, Alice, I'm Latisha. Would you sign your autograph for my kids?" asked a round-faced African American woman, holding out paper and pen. "Your lawyer told us that you wrote for Nickelodeon television shows, and my children love Nickelodeon. Thank you. Make two of them, please, or they'll fight over it. Tanisha and Tyrell, T-Y-R-E-L-L. The way your lawyer talked about you, you were right to fight this case for your daughter and not just let them stupid-ass doctors do what they want and take no responsibility. This trial was an act of love, from you to your daughter, that's for sure. Now you go home and you love that little girl of yours. I'm goin' home and tellin' my kids that I am proud of the service I performed today. Like Judge Snow said, it was because of us being out here that your daughter got what she needs. Thank you for the autographs, and God bless you."

Twelve jurors and two alternates, in a celebratory mood, their jury duty fulfilled, filled pockets and pocketbooks with Halloween candy till the bowl was empty, by order of the judge.

Nine days later, Julia aced her Hebrew Torah reading and enthralled her audience with her provocative speech on The Binding of Isaac. Eliana's babysitter chased her through the aisles and under the seats, and finally carried her outside to the lobby when she got too distracting. When the bat mitzvah service was over, everyone walked two blocks from the synagogue to the restaurant, for a joyful celebration and spicy Turkish buffet, with optional burgers and fries for Julia and her friends. Mahmood took care of everything.

Epilogue

I have two daughters.

One is tall and sturdy, earthbound. Our Rock of Gibraltar, steady as she goes.

The other is short and slight, of the air, lightning quick. Unpredictable and moody.

Julia wears size eleven extra wide shoes. Firmly planted on the ground, she knows where she stands.

Eliana, at age seven, still wears toddler-sized shoes, the right foot two sizes smaller than the left. She is featherweight. Her right foot doesn't quite reach the ground, so she flies above it, running faster than imagination, jumping intrepidly from her bed to Julia's, scampering up the rocks in Central Park.

Julia at sixteen is calm and centered, even-keeled. Her friends come to her for advice, even about things she knows nothing about. She is confident and reliable.

Eliana is quicksilver in temperament. Falls in and out of love with toys and friends, has crushes, has asked three different boys on three Valentine's Days, "Are you my secret admirer?" When the baffled boys ask back, "What's that?" she explains, "It means you love someone but you don't want them to know it." Each boy has thoughtfully stared at his feet for a moment, then nodded and agreed, "Yeah," whereupon Eliana understands that he is no longer what he just admitted he was. A secret admirer lasts only as long as the secret, and once the secret is revealed, it is time to cultivate another secret admirer or secretly admired.

Days of Awe

It is Erev Rosh Hashanah, 2006.

It is the first year since 1999 that it falls on a Friday. Again, it is early, four days after Labor Day. Again, it's a brilliant, sunny day. I walk to Central Park and Turtle Pond—redwing blackbirds perch on cattails, a white heron fishes on the far shore, seven turtles line up on a log, reaching for the afternoon's last rays of sun, the pond framed by weeping willows, the willows framed by the Manhattan skyline, the skyline framed by the cloudless blue sky.

I walk home and start to write.

What I Know

- Eliana is a second-grader with an awesome sense of humor.
- Julia is a high school junior, looking at colleges.
- She wants to find her birth mother some day.
- Eliana is now Eliana's legal name.
- Michael has a new career in corporate communications.
- We're out of debt.

- Eliana takes a growth hormone shot every night and is growing well.
- She wears a two-inch lift on her right shoe, and will probably have the first of two complicated leg-lengthening surgeries in a year.
- I've stopped taking antidepressants and am relieved that I'm no longer emotionally anaesthetized by a drug.
- Michael and I have a new bed.
- We're a family of four with four last names.
- After seven years of writer's block, I start to write. Unexpectedly. Urgently. I write as fast as I can, without telling anybody. For fear that I'll stop. For fear that the Evil Eye will catch up with me.
- *Tuh! Tuh! Tuh!*

On Yom Kippur, I decide to take Eliana to the afternoon children's service. She has chosen her fanciest dress, with a red velvet bodice and an ankle-length gold chiffon skirt, and her gold party shoes. The dress is too fancy for synagogue, but what the heck, she loves wearing it.

"Can I bring my scooter?"

"Sure. Why not?"

"Where are we going again?"

I hesitate. Last year's children's service was a mob scene, and Eliana is overwhelmed by crowds. "Your choice. We can either go to synagogue like we did last year. Or we can climb the rocks in Central Park and we'll have our own Yom Kippur service, just the two of us."

"Central Park! Central Park! Can I get a hot dog?"

Eliana rides her scooter toward Central Park. In her long velvet dress and gold party shoes, people stop to stare and smile at the incongruous sight of a little girl in a ball gown riding a scooter, and then glance down curiously at the two-inch lift on her right shoe.

She zigs and zags expertly through the crowded sidewalks, oblivious to the attention she attracts. My beautiful, asymmetrical little girl, negotiating her imaginary slalom course. We stop at the hot dog stand in front of the Museum of Natural History.

Hot dog in one hand, she glides down the hill into Central Park. We stash the scooter and climb the rocks. Overlooking the lake, ringed by trees just beginning to change color, she eats her hot dog, while I give her the Cliffs Notes version of Yom Kippur.

We reflect on the past year, the things we might learn from and do differently next time. We talk about our wishes for next year. We think of anyone who has made us angry in the past year and we talk about forgiving them, about forgiving ourselves. I tell her about the Book of Life.

She takes a bite of her hot dog, drips ketchup on her velvet dress.

"Mom, do you believe in God?"

"I don't know."

"That's impossible. How can you not know?"

"I don't know. I've always felt that way."

"Really? That's exactly the way I feel. I thought I was the only one in the whole world who felt that way."

"Nope, there are at least two of us."

And yet,

I chose her name,

Eliana—"My God has answered me."

I still don't know which one of us is the "me."

Maybe "me" is both of us—a symmetry, a palindrome, Eliana and I mirroring each other. "I don't know if I believe in God, but somehow . . ."

My question or hers was answered. What question?

I don't know if I believe in God.

I didn't think I wanted this—this being born; this giving birth.

I don't remember asking to be here with you. But somehow we ended up here on top of the rocks together.

The sky is impossibly blue.

Eliana finishes her hot dog.

She lies down with her head in my lap.

"My God has answered me."

Acknowledgments

Thanks above all to my editor, Carole DeSanti, for her wise edits and insights, and to my extraordinary agent, Sally Wofford-Girand, for believing in my book and for so quickly finding a wonderful home for it. Much gratitude to Kristin Spang at Viking, and to Melissa Sarver at Brick House Literary Agents, for their invaluable help and great patience.

Deep gratitude and love to my smart, talented friends—Patty McCormick, Melissa Kraft, Kathy Mendeloff, Jackie Reingold, Ricki Rosen, Susan Stephen, and Diane Umansky—who generously read the manuscript when I was still scared to show it to anybody, and who persuaded me that it was a book people would want to read; with special thanks to Patty, whose encouragement gave me the courage to begin writing the story, and who proved herself a brilliant matchmaker by introducing the book to my agent.

I want to thank my New School students, whose beautiful and resonant words I've quoted (I've changed their names in the book to protect their privacy); with gratitude to and in memory of Dani Athena Nikas.

My tremendous affection and thanks to my sisters and best friends, Madeline Cohen and Jennifer Cohen, and to my father Ira Cohen, for their constant love and encouragement. In fond memory of my mother, Louise Giventer Cohen.

My deepest gratitude to my beloved and loving family, for taking this life journey together and for allowing me to share our story—my husband, Michael, soul mate in joyful times and dark times, as well as my thoughtful literary adviser; and my two beautiful daughters, Julia and Eliana, who never cease to amaze and inspire me, whom I love more than anything in the world.